PRAISE FOR *BLOOM*

"*Dr. Carrasco is a bright light in the world of functional medi-cine. She leverages the most forward-minded clinical research combined with a fresh perspective on how compassionate self-care, nourishment, and natural medicine can bring one back to a state of sustainable wholeness.*"

—MARK HYMAN, M.D.
TEN-TIME #1 *NEW YORK TIMES* BESTSELLING
AUTHOR AND MEDICAL DIRECTOR AT CLEVELAND
CLINIC'S CENTER FOR FUNCTIONAL MEDICINE

"*In Bloom, Dr. Carrasco has outlined exactly what it takes for women to overcome modern health challenges while nurturing a conscious attitude of growth, self-care, and compassion.*"

—IZABELLA WENTZ, PHARMD, FASCP
#1 *NEW YORK TIMES* BESTSELLING AUTHOR
OF *HASHIMOTO'S PROTOCOL*

"*Bloom demystifies the world of nutrition, detoxification, and functional medicine while providing a compassionate template for women to take back control of their health and live their lives with meaning and joy.*"

"*Are you stressed, tired, sick, hopeless, and dragging through each day? Then let this remarkable book show you the road back to a healthy and joy-filled life. Bloom's seven simple and powerful steps will empower you to regain your energy, heal your body, and rekindle your "spark." Filled with wisdom and compassion, this book is a must for any woman who wants to truly live rather than merely survive.*"

"*Dr. Alex invites you to explore your infinite potential as a woman! Bloom gives women proven and effective strategies to create amazing energy, resiliency to life's stress, and tools to raise the vibrancy of their spirit to truly flourish.*"

"Dr. Carrasco's approach to compassionate healing, along with her meticulous research and easy-to-follow advice on detoxification, nutrition, and functional medicine, makes this an instant classic for health-conscious women."

—DR. V. DESAULNIERS
BEST-SELLING AUTHOR AND FOUNDER OF BREAST CANCER
CONQUEROR AND THE 7 ESSENTIALS SYSTEM

"This is the book I wish I had read when I was a young mom. In Bloom Dr. Alex gets to the heart of women's greatest fears and health challenges by offering seven powerfully practical steps to reclaim your health, sanity, and spark for living. All women can benefit from the wisdom and strategies this book offers, and I look forward to recommending it to my patients."

—NICOLE BEURKENS, PHD, CNS
LICENSED PSYCHOLOGIST AND BOARD-
CERTIFIED NUTRITION SPECIALIST

"Dr. Carrasco has created a complete guide to harnessing the power of integrative medicine for the modern woman. Bloom shows readers, specifically busy, stressed-out women, how to hit the reset button on their physical, emotional, and spiritual health, and how to cultivate vitality for the long run. This will be recommended reading for all of my patients."

—SHAWN TASSONE, MD, PHD
AUTHOR OF SPIRITUAL PREGNANCY: DEVELOP, NURTURE,
AND EMBRACE THE JOURNEY TO MOTHERHOOD

"Dr. Alex's compassionate and artful seven-step healing process guides readers on a practical journey to root out and resolve unwanted ailments, while creating an abundant reservoir of health for the future."

—ANTHONY YOUN, MD
AMERICA'S HOLISTIC PLASTIC SURGEON AND
BEST-SELLING AUTHOR OF *THE AGE FIX*

"Dr. Carrasco's Bloom provides inspiring and insightful science-based solutions to help you find true health—mind, body, and spirit. It's a must-read!"

—ANN SHIPPY, MD
FUNCTIONAL-MEDICINE PHYSICIAN

"*Bloom* is a refreshing and informative read that provides the modern woman with an essential mix of education, inspiration, and tools to reignite her lost desires and empower herself back to a true and lasting state of optimal health and well-being. Dr. Carrasco does an amazing job structuring this book to uncover hidden ailments to support women at every phase of their healing journey."

—DR. MARIZA SNYDER
BEST-SELLING AUTHOR OF
SMART MOM'S GUIDE TO ESSENTIAL OILS

BLOOM

Bloom

7 Steps to Reclaim Your Health,
Cultivate Your Desires & Reignite Your Spark

Alejandra Carrasco, MD

This publication contains the opinions and ideas of the author. It is intended to provide helpful and informative material on the subjects addressed in the publication. It is sold with the understanding that the author is not engaged in rendering medical, health, psychological, or any other kind of professional services in the book. If the reader requires personal medical, health, or other assistance or advice, a competent professional should be consulted.

The author specifically disclaims all responsibility for any liability, loss, or risk, personal or otherwise, that is incurred as a consequence, directly or indirectly, of the use and application of the contents of this book.

BLOOM

7 Steps to Reclaim Your Health, Cultivate
Your Desires & Reignite Your Spark

ISBN   978-1-61961-734-6   *Paperback*

        978-1-61961-735-3   *Ebook*

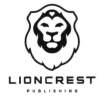

LIONCREST
PUBLISHING

For Danny—whose love and devotion nourishes me profoundly.

*For Mami and Papi—whose love and care has
given me deep and enduring roots.*

*And for Camila and Lucho—whose love and affection
inspire me to live my life in full bloom.*

Contents

Introduction

———

Once upon a time, there were two best friends who each decided to start a garden.

The first friend worked a demanding job, had two children to take care of, and not a lot of time for herself. Eager to see the fruits of her labor, she took the modern route.

She paid landscapers to dig up a random garden plot in the backyard, bought pre-planted seedlings from the big box store, a huge bag of fertilizer-infused drought-resistant potting soil, pesticides, weed killer, and quickly threw everything into the ground as fast as she could.

She watered when she thought about it, applied weed killer once a week, sprayed pesticides at the first sign of a bug, and waited for her garden to grow.

We'll call her "the hurried gardener."

The second friend also worked a demanding job, took care of two children, and had very little time. She decided to fully embrace the gardening process as a stress-relieving exercise; she included her children, and took the more sustainable route.

She carefully chose a plot of land with just enough sun and protection from the elements, she had her soil tested, so she knew how to best nourish it; she sourced out hardy, heirloom seeds and started them indoors; she amended her soil with organic compost, patiently "hardened" her seedlings before transplanting outdoors; and finally, she planted them into the rich soil following the season's last frost. Then, she and her children took turns mulching, watering, pulling weeds by hand, pruning branches, and even singing to their plants while they patiently waited for them to grow.

We'll call her "the mindful gardener."

The hurried gardener's garden grew quickly. However, the plants were sporadic in size and hardiness; their roots were shallow; pests were a constant problem; the fruits and vegetables looked nice but lacked flavor; and when the first big storm came, it uprooted nearly all the plants. The hurried gardener was left defeated, with little to show for her efforts.

The mindful gardener's garden required more effort and took a little longer to grow. With her tender love, patience, and care, the garden was well nourished, and the blooms, fruits, and vegetables grew strong, resilient, and produced the most intensely pleasing flavors, colors, and aromas.

What's more, the garden provided a much-needed sanctuary for her. A quiet, beautiful place to slow down, be present, and reconnect with herself and her children as she cared for the earth.

When autumn came, the hurried gardener felt regret, for she had only a muddy, weed-ridden plot of soil left. Her garden was spent.

Meanwhile, the mindful gardener carefully gathered all the seeds from her remaining plants to use the following year and had more than enough seed left to share the precious gifts of her little garden with her friend and the greater world.

HOW DOES *YOUR* GARDEN GROW?

Most of us who live in the real world—working, raising kids with little support, and chasing dreams—are more likely to identify with the "hurried gardener." Imagine for a moment *you* are the mindful gardener, and *you* are standing in your beautiful garden.

What does your garden look like?

What fruits, vegetables, and flowers do you see and smell?

How does it feel to stand in the middle of the beautiful, blooming, vibrant garden that you created and tended?

The story of the two gardeners is an analogy for the rest of this book. You, the reader, are both the gardener (hurried or mindful) and the garden of your own level of health, vitality, and happiness.

So, how does your garden grow?

If at this moment you identify with the hurried gardener, or you wince at the thought of gardening altogether, FEAR NOT and KEEP READING because this book was written for you. Over the next few chapters, I will guide you through the same seven-step process I have used with thousands of patients to help them get to the root of their health issues and establish a clear path to lifelong well-being.

This book was not written for one particular condition or ailment, nor does it offer a fixed "protocol" for reclaiming health. Rather, it is structured so anyone at any phase in their health journey can use it to uncover hidden ailments, pull them out by the root, and get on with living a vibrant life.

This book was built around comparisons to gardening for a reason: I was inspired to write it when I started my own garden, because in doing so I realized just how close an analogy it is to the state of the modern woman's health.

Here's how we will work together using these seven steps to reclaim your health, cultivate your desires, and reignite your spark.

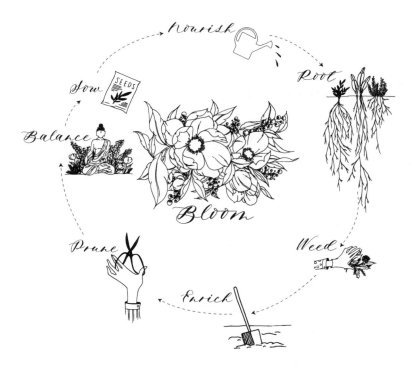

Before we begin our steps and journey together, you will be invited to give yourself official, signed permission to go through the Bloom process. We will also discuss how to open your mind to embrace expansion, growth, and self-compassion, which will fuel the healing process ahead.

Once we have gotten your head and heart in the game (so to speak), we will move on to Step 1: SOW.

This first step takes you through a specific exercise to identify and own your core desires for your health and life—which I call "seeds." These will be different for everyone and will form the basis, purpose, and desired outcome of your Bloom journey. Once we have isolated those unique seeds of desire, we will "sow" or manifest them by uncovering the big "Why" behind those desires, setting goals, and putting your personal health plan in place. This step is the most important in the entire process, as it establishes the framework from which you will build upon in your journey to achieving full Bloom.

Now that you have an actionable plan in place, we will move on to Step 2: NOURISH.

This second step shows you how to nourish yourself by making the right food choices for your individual biology and current state of health. You will learn exactly how to nurture your personal earth by identifying energy-sapping food sensitivities, optimizing nutrient intake, choosing the right supplements, and increasing your consumption of the little-known "primary foods." By taking the time to nourish yourself in this step—body, mind, and spirit—you prepare your body to heal fully in the steps ahead.

With your individual nourishment strategy in place, we will continue along the garden path to Step 3: ROOT.

In this step, you will learn how to establish strong, deep roots and become grounded by switching your nervous system response to "calm," resetting your sleep cycle, and reconnecting to yourself, and others, spiritually. By embracing this step fully, you will establish an unshakeable inner strength and stability you would have not thought possible.

With your roots firmly established, we move into new territory in Step 4: WEED.

This step goes in-depth by teaching you exactly how to find and weed out the numerous insidious toxins in your food, home, environment, and relationships that quietly degrade your health. This is a crucial step in reducing body burden and overcoming many puzzling health issues.

Now that you have learned to weed your garden effectively, you are ready for Step 5: ENRICH.

This fifth step is profound as it shows you how to identify and heal common gut-health issues using food, lab work, and natural remedies. Gut-health abnormalities are at the heart of many chronic conditions plaguing women, such as autoimmune disease and mood disorders. This one step alone, if taken seriously, will help you restore immunity, optimize nutrient absorption, stabilize your mood, and prevent a cascade of future health issues.

In Step 6: PRUNE, we will work on trimming back the overgrowth surrounding your symptoms.

In this step, we will determine if you would benefit from partnering with a functional medicine physician. You will also learn about the most common underdiagnosed health issues, subclinical, and clinical conditions affecting women, and exactly which advanced lab tests will help your new doctor identify them. Step 6 will help you get unstuck, over the hump, or it will arm you with the information you need to establish a reputable healthcare team that can help you nip any future conditions in the bud.

With the overgrowth pruned and your desired health outcomes in sight, we move confidently into our final step together, Step 7: BALANCE.

This last step shows you how to create *resiliency* in your

health, so you can weather the inevitable storms of life and health. You will learn how to use mindfulness, energy healing, and the power of nature to stay strong, no matter what life throws at you, plus how to return to these seven steps any time you need to reset a specific area of your health and well-being.

Finally, after all seven steps are completed, we will take a moment to reflect on all you have done to come to this point of full Bloom, and how you can harvest your seeds of health and share them with the greater world.

How do I know this seven-step process can work for you?

Because, as a physician, I have used these same seven steps as guiding principles to treat hundreds of patients with thousands of symptoms in my own integrative functional medicine practice—many of whom you will meet in the coming chapters. That is the beauty of this process, it does not discriminate based on your age, level of health, or diagnosis; rather, its application and results are universal and can be tailored to meet your needs within life's ever-changing seasons.

Before we get started, let me tell you a bit about my harrowing journey from health- train-wreck-medical-student to integrative-medicine-specialist, and how the "Bloom" process came to be.

I'm Alejandra Carrasco, M.D. or "Dr. Alex" as my patients call me. I'm a mother of two young children, wife and partner to my soulmate, and a board-certified medical doctor practicing integrative and functional medicine.

In the integrative functional medicine model, we seek to treat the whole person by uncovering the root cause of illness, not just masking the symptoms. To do this, we rely on a systems-based approach to every patient, which includes a lengthy intake and history, advanced laboratory testing, and a heavy reliance on integrative therapies such as functional nutrition, pharmaceutical grade nutritional supplementation, herbal medicine, and mind-body healing.

I often compare the goal of integrative functional medicine to that of treating a splinter: if you get a big, painful splinter in your foot you're not going to treat it with painkillers and hope it goes away, you're going to remove the splinter. Functional medicine follows the same practical course—treat the cause, not the symptoms.

The path to my current method, however, was neither straight nor smooth. I used to be the mirror image of the "hurried gardener," complete with a debilitating bill of health to boot.

My whole life, I aspired to be a doctor. It was like a spiritual calling, and since there were no doctors in my family, I was forging a new path. It was an exciting, purposeful, and incredibly *stressful* journey that consumed my childhood, teen, and young adult years.

After years of test-stress, completing undergrad, and passing the MCAT, my hard work paid off, and I finally got into medical school. My excitement turned to anxiety as I was introduced to the brutal realities of medical school. I went from a small, forward-thinking, liberal arts university, to eighteen-hour days of studying in an incredibly competitive, cold, and institutional environment. It sent my stress levels through the roof, but I adapted and carried on.

Then, after two years of grueling work, I reached the Holy Grail: seeing patients. This was the moment I had waited for my whole life, but things went downhill fast.

Almost overnight, I developed full-blown panic attacks that struck anywhere—during rounds at the hospital, in the middle of church, at dinner with friends—severe irritable bowel syndrome that reared its ugly head at the worst possible times, migraine headaches, and extreme fatigue.

It hit me like a ton of bricks, and left me scrambling from doctor to doctor, getting test after test, CT scans, EKGs, etc., with little more insight than: "Your tests are normal. You must be stressed. Here are a bunch of prescriptions you can start taking."

Obviously, that wasn't the answer I was looking for. Though I was relieved everything appeared "normal," I didn't *feel* normal, and I didn't know how to fix any of my symptoms.

On top of it all, I experienced crushing feelings of shame and helplessness. I had made it all this way and sacrificed so much, only to be knocked off my game by mysterious ailments dismissed by the medical professionals I looked up to. Plus, I was training to be a doctor, for God's sake. I even practiced yoga and ate organic food—what patient in their right mind would want to take advice from a doctor in such poor health?

However, one thing those specialists told me hit home—*I was stressed*. Stressed to the max, and I had been stressed as long as I could remember. I had been chased by the proverbial lion for way too long and my body was finally breaking down.

Fortunately, that's when I met Sister Alice—a seventy-year-old Catholic nun who enthusiastically studied Buddhism, Kabbalah, and many of the different mystical practices, in addition to Catholic doctrine. She became my lifeboat. She taught me how to use meditation and centering prayer to take the edge off my anxiety and control my panic attacks. This got me through that third year in medical school.

Then, as I went into my fourth year, I was fortunate to do a rotation at Dr. Andrew Weil's Arizona Center for Integrative Medicine at the University of Arizona. It was a real education in botanical medicine, nutrition, bodywork, acupuncture, energy medicine, and all the different forms of healing practiced throughout the world.

As I learned about these ancient healing practices, I couldn't help but wonder why we didn't use these tools in the conventional medical model. When I asked Dr. Weil, "Why are we stuck in this paradigm? Why do we act as if everything is so separate?" He replied, to paraphrase, that "Integrative medicine is just good medicine. We shouldn't have to separate it from conventional medicine. Unfortunately, given the way the system is built, that's just what we must do."

My time in Arizona was therapeutic on so many levels, and after graduation, my anxiety had nearly disappeared, but I continued to suffer from intense migraines and irritable bowel syndrome. That's when I met Dr. Mark Hyman, currently the medical director of the Cleveland Clinic's Center for Functional Medicine, at a conference.

I had no idea who he was at the time, but he spoke about the science and systems of functional medicine in a way never presented to me in medical school. I knew I had to connect with him, so I approached him after his lecture, and he graciously gave me his email address. We corresponded about my health issues, and on his advice, I went gluten-free, dairy-free, and off processed foods. I must admit, after all my years of training in conventional and integrative medicine, I didn't expect a miracle from this, but that's exactly what I got.

Within two weeks, my bowels were normal for the first time in two years, and my migraines were much better too. I was blown away. It had taken me two years to get a handle on any of my own issues, and within two weeks, they were nearly gone. I had not encountered anyone treating people as Dr. Hyman had suggested in the conventional medical world. That was when I knew I would follow the functional medicine path.

After completing a family medicine residency and taking a soul-sucking job in urgent care (which required me to dole out unnecessary amounts of antibiotics and other prescriptions every day), I knew I had to start my own functional medicine practice. I had to practice medicine in a way that was aligned with my soul.

That's how I got here. Now, every day since 2012, I help patients get to the root cause of their health issues and heal themselves—body, mind, and spirit—using a purely integrative and functional medicine approach. Plus, my own health has bloomed; no more panic attacks, anxiety, or IBS. I am fulfilling my purpose, and in honoring that, I could heal myself.

I know this book can help you do the same.

WHO IS THIS BOOK FOR?

This book was written for the stressed out, the sleepless, the hormonal, the moody, the exhausted, the uninspired-ready-to-be-inspired, the overweight—be it ten pounds or one hundred pounds—the person who knows something is wrong even when their doctor says they are "normal," and the "spent."

It was written specifically for women—mothers, daughters, aunts, and grandmothers who have lost touch with themselves and their health, and are tired of feeling sick, fatigued, and stuck just "surviving" at life.

If you are ready to stop "surviving" and start living your life in full Bloom, then step through the garden gate, and let's get started.

CHAPTER 1

Preparing the Soil: Permission and Attitude

———

YOUR PERMISSION SLIP TO HEALTH

Flip the Switch!

A woman found herself in the middle of a pitch-black room. She prayed, cried, and begged for the light to turn on.

"Please God," she called. "Please turn the light on. I don't want to be in the dark."

The light never turned on. She kept praying and crying out, and yet it remained dark.

After some time, an angel appeared before her and said, "God hears your heartfelt prayers, but is wondering why you don't just stand up and flip the switch on the wall."

The woman replied, "Oh—I didn't realize I could."

I see this exact story played out every single day in my practice. A patient comes to me distraught, shamed, and feeling powerless, after having their health concerns dismissed by the conventional medical system.

They are typically told, "All your tests are normal, it must be stress. Here's a prescription for anti-anxiety pills and sleep meds."

The great news is we have the power to flip on that proverbial light switch—to keep searching for answers, to do our own research (like reading this book), to listen to our bodies and intuition, and to find the right healthcare providers to help us reclaim our health. We all have the power; all we must do to flip the switch is to STOP giving our power away.

As mentioned in the introduction, before we can get started on the seven steps to reclaiming your health, cultivating your desires, and reigniting your spark, we must do a little preliminary work to prepare your soil for what is to come.

This means becoming aware of how you take care of yourself, and how you don't.

When I ask my patients how they take care of themselves on their first visit, nearly all of them stare at me blankly, and then we engage in a dialogue like this:

The patient says, "What do you mean?"

I explain, "Well, how do you nurture yourself? What do you do that brings you joy? What do you do for self-care? What hobbies do you have? What dreams do you have for yourself?"

Then, after laughing, scowling, or thinking hard, they answer something like, "Gosh—no one has asked me in such a long time. After I got married/started a demanding career/became a mom, all those things took a back seat. Honestly, I feel like I just can't do those things anymore. I have too many tasks to complete, other people to take care of, and responsibilities to fulfill. All that taking-care-of-me stuff feels selfish."

There it is. The dreaded "s" word when it comes to women's health and happiness: "selfish." Our mothers felt it, our grandmothers felt it, but I would wager no generation feels it quite so profoundly as the busy, stressed, and isolated working moms of twenty-first century America.

Well, here's the thing: "All that taking-care-of-me stuff" is not selfish—it's *essential*. If my experience as a doctor and former health-train-wreck has taught me anything, it's this: If *you* aren't well cared for, then you can't share your gifts with others effectively. If you're not able to share your gifts, you will feel empty, unfulfilled, and burnt out, because a huge part of fulfilling our life's purpose comes down to our ability to effectively share our gifts and sow and grow our seeds.

Too often, due to cultural, family, or self-imposed expectations, we think we must pour ourselves out completely—into our work and others—to give generously. If you pour everything out, what is left for you? How do you refill your cup?

Just like in the story of the hurried gardener or my story of med-school burnout, you can't give what you don't have. If you keep pouring yourself out without refilling your cup, eventually you will have nothing left to give, and your health will suffer. You deserve to live a healthy, joyful, and deeply satisfying life, but you've got to give yourself the opportunity to do so. If you want to get better, have more energy, feel happy and fulfilled, and rediscover what "normal" should feel like, you need to give yourself *permission* to take care of yourself, to amend and prepare your personal soil for growth in a profound way.

What does it mean to give yourself permission in the context of this book? Imagine you are preparing a space for your garden plot, choosing the right location with enough sun and space for the plants to grow and enough protection from the elements. Likewise, as you begin this journey, I want you to give yourself the freedom, time, and space to follow these seven guiding principles. Even if some of the work feels indulgent or uncomfortable, you must prepare mental space for growth and expansion.

How much time will you need to dedicate to this process? That is up to you, as I understand everyone's circumstances and health issues are different. However, I would recommend you commit to reading one chapter a day, and implementing at least one to three of the recommendations therein. Depending upon how fast you read (and this book was designed for skimmers and detailed-readers alike), that could take up to thirty minutes a day for reading, and additional time to implement the recommendations. If you wish to read faster, be my guest. If you want to see real changes in your health, you must implement what you learn.

Remember when you were a child, and a responsible adult

signed your permission slips for different school activities? Well, now YOU are the responsible adult, and I want you to sign the permission slip below and commit to allowing yourself the time and space to reclaim your health and happiness.

Sign this permission slip and give yourself the gift of permission.

I, _____, give myself permission to prepare the space and time to apply these seven steps to reclaim my health, cultivate my desires, and reignite my spark. I give myself permission to come into full BLOOM.

Date:

Signature:

CULTIVATING AN ATTITUDE OF HEALTH— PERFECTION OR EXPANSION

Now that you have given yourself permission to go through this process (huge congrats!), it's time to talk about how attitude, or our overall beliefs about health and healing, can affect this seven-step process.

When it comes to health, there are essentially two attitudes dominating the conversation.

The first is a perfectionist attitude. The perfectionist attitude thrives in a rigid frame of mind, avoiding failure at all costs (because it is seen as a huge weakness), and seeking a fixed idea of perfection as their ultimate goal. The perfectionist is focused on the end result only, and therefore misses out on what could be gained through adapting to the natural ebbs and flows of a process.

The second is an attitude of expansion. The expansive attitude focuses more on growth and progress than achieving perfection. Those who adopt and cultivate this attitude do not fear failure, because they know setbacks can wind up being great blessings if they are willing to learn and grow from them.

It is critical you realize the importance of adopting an attitude of expansion with respect to this process, because cultivating true and lasting health is not a rigid process or destination. Rather, like a garden, it goes through cycles unique to the individual's desires, goals, circumstances, limitations, capabilities, and season of life. Perfection is not the goal.

The great news is, if you suspect you have been living with a perfectionist attitude, you can easily switch to an expansive attitude with very little effort. Here's how to cultivate the new soil of an expansive attitude:

- When faced with a challenge, embrace it and view it as an opportunity to grow.
- Make a concerted effort to embrace change, because that effort will lead to growth. It may not feel comfortable at first, but building up an expansive attitude is like building a muscle—you must train it and strengthen it.
- Remember that mistakes are opportunities to learn. They are just data points that can help you reverse your course into a more positive direction.

To summarize, your attitude toward health and growth is not set in stone, and that is great news for all of us, because, regardless of our past, we can all adopt expansive attitudes. If you find yourself slipping back into a perfectionist attitude or state of mind at any time during this process, just return to this chapter and repeat this exercise as many times as you need to. You will get there because the very nature of life is to EXPAND and GROW.

See, prepping your soil wasn't so hard, was it? You didn't even have to get your hands dirty. Next, we will officially start with our first step in the Bloom journey by creating your health goals and sowing your seeds of intention, desire, and compassion.

Preparing the Soil Action Steps:

1.   What is your attitude or frame of mind when it comes to your current state of health? Perfectionist or expansive? Complete the exercise at nourishmedicine.com/bloomresources to start achieving a more consistent attitude of expansion.

2.   Sign your permission slip—download this at nourishmedicine.com/bloomresources —hang it up, take a picture of it.

3.   Write down one thing (besides reading this book) you will do to care for yourself this week. Some ideas: take an Epsom salt bath, meditate for ten minutes, give yourself a facial, pick up an old hobby you used to enjoy, or spend time with a girlfriend (no kids allowed).

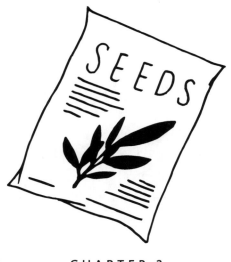

Step 1: SOW—Intention, Desire, and Compassion for Self

EVERY PLANT, TREE, AND BLOSSOM STARTS AS A SEED

Now that you have prepared your soil by giving yourself permission to undergo this process and switch to an attitude of expansion, it's time for Step 1: Sowing Your

Seeds—which are the specific desires and intentions you hold for your health.

Even before I gardened, seeds had always fascinated me. These teeny embryonic plants are chock full of dormant potential but will only awaken when given the ideal environment and the right amount of tending and care. Likewise, your metaphorical seeds of desire and intention will sprout, grow, bloom, fruit, and flourish as you provide them with the proper consideration, attention, and care.

As you sow, so shall you reap, and that is what this step is all about: selecting the seeds you wish to sow and creating the perfect environment for them to be planted, so they can awaken, grow, and bloom.

To begin this step, I will take you through a series of mini-steps to help you choose exactly what "seeds" you want to sow in your life. This seed selection process is a crucial first step in getting the health outcomes you want in your life, so do not skip it.

THE PROCESS OF INTENTION

The process of intention is a concept that describes the steps that will take you from intention and desire (SOWing seeds) to our ultimate outcome: health (BLOOM).

The first mini-step starts by defining your *overall* desires.

- How do you want to *feel* in your life?
    - Happy?
    - Joyful?
    - Calm?
    - Inspired?
    - Free?
- What are your specific desires for your *health*?
    - What do you want to change about your health?
    - Do you want to stop feeling so tired all the time?
    - Do you want better digestion?
    - More stable mood?
    - To lose weight?
    - To sleep better? Etc.

The second mini-step is to create an intention. Now if the word "intention" drums up images of new age gurus (or "enlightened" CEOs) sitting around a circle repeating positive affirmations, keep in mind an intention is just the goal, aim, or purpose you set to accomplish; or if you're the kind of person who lives to manifest your intentions, then by all means start manifesting!

In the third mini-step, it's time to act to achieve your intention/goal. In the Bloom process, this may mean cleaning up your diet, eliminating toxic influences in your life, and creating a daily self-care regime (more on this to come).

The fruits of your actions are your outcome. In this case, your outcome may be more energy, resolution of a chronic condition, inner peace, weight loss, or a renewed confidence in your ability to care for yourself.

The seven steps outlined in this book follow the process of intention:

- Define your desires and create specific intentions (SOW—as you will today).
- Take strategic actions (NOURISH, ROOT, WEED, ENRICH, PRUNE).
- Finally, enjoy your outcome (BLOOM).

Though the principle is simple, it is important to understand the process, so we can create clarity around your desires, intentions, and actions as we move through these seven steps together.

Now, let's start by selecting your *Seeds of Desire*.

Desires are the things you wish for yourself and for your life—and more importantly, the ways in which you want to feel.

To help you select your Seeds of Desire, I have created a Seed Word Box below. As you browse through these Seed Words, I want you to think about the positive outcomes they suggest. Which ones resonate with you in relation to your health and life goals? Do you wish for any of these things to manifest in your life? Put a checkmark next to the words that resonate with you (and don't worry about checking off too many, we will whittle it down in the next section).

Seed Words

- abundance
- adventure
- balance
- beauty (inner)
- beauty (outer)
- cheer
- clarity
- compassion
- connection
- creativity
- delight
- desire
- empowerment
- energy
- enthusiasm
- expansiveness
- femininity
- forgiveness, self and others
- freedom

- groundedness
- happiness
- healing
- health
- hope
- imagination
- inspiration
- lightheartedness
- love/loved/loving
- magic
- nourishment
- pain-free
- peace
- pleasure
- purpose
- radiant
- receptiveness
- regeneration
- relaxation
- restoration
- rootedness
- satisfaction
- spontaneity
- strength
- tranquility
- transformation
- understanding
- unity
- vibrancy
- vitality
- warmth
- wellness
- wisdom
- worthiness
- youthfulness

Now that you have checked off your Seed Words, it's time to narrow them down to your top three. These are the desires we will focus on as we begin this journey together. These are the three things you want to *feel* most of all in your life and health.

These core desires are your "seeds," and they are precious, so take your time in selecting them.

Write them down below or using the downloadable form provided at the end of this chapter on the Bloom Resources website.

Seeds:

1.

2.

3.

If you need more help pinning down your top three, see the resources section at the end of this chapter for a special meditation to zero in on your core desires.

YOUR BIG WHY

Nice work narrowing down the list to your top three seeds. Now that you have them, I want you to think about Why you want to feel this way. Defining your Why is crucial for motivation, purpose, and direction throughout the Bloom journey, which will make this process—or any process in life—easier.

Grab your journal or in the space below write down why you want to feel this way based on your Seed Words/core desires. To help you get in the flow, I suggest using the "so that" method.

For example:

1. Seed Word: Joyful: I want to feel joyful, so that I will be a better parent and spouse, and can approach my life with more enthusiasm.
2. Seed Word: Energetic: I want to feel energetic, so that I can play with my kids and make memories with them.
3. Seed Word: Forgiveness: I want to feel forgiveness, so that I can experience more love and forgiveness in my life.

Now it's your turn, go:

1.

2.

3.

I know self-care and self-analysis aren't always the most natural or comfortable things in the world, but by completing these exercises you are well on your way to cultivating a happier and healthier you.

If, like many others, you are struggling with your big Whys, try returning to the first exercise to make sure you have selected the seeds you truly desire. If you are certain you have chosen the right seeds but can't flesh out the Whys behind them, you can try one of two options:

- Option 1: Look at it another way and ask yourself: "How will this positively affect other people (your spouse, partner, children, friends, etc.) in my life?"
- Option 2: Check out the resources section at the end of this chapter to help you discover your Whys.

PEELING BACK THE ONION LAYERS OF "WHY"

Natalie came to my practice at the end of her rope. At the ripe old age of thirty-one, she suffered from a plethora of mysterious symptoms with no conclusive diagnosis in sight.

She was exhausted, her hair was falling out, she had digestive distress, panic attacks, trouble focusing, unexplained weight gain, and terrible joint pain. She was overwhelmed, underserved by her doctors, and didn't know how to make sense of her baffling symptoms. We did a thorough intake and history, ordered some lab tests, and started prioritizing by figuring out what changes she desired most in her health and life (her seeds) and *Why* she desired those changes.

At first, the exercise was difficult and a bit awkward for her; but as we went through it together, she discovered what she wanted and needed. First and foremost was more energy, so she could have the resolve to work on the rest of her health issues. Next, she desired to get her digestion back on track, so she could eliminate those embarrassing trips to the bathroom and find joy in eating and socializing again—which in turn would help with her weight gain. Finally, she wanted to get her panic attacks under control, so she could feel strength in herself again. So, Natalie's seeds were: energy, joy, and strength.

The wonderful thing about Natalie's story, and most others, is—as she planted and nourished these seeds of intention—most of her other symptoms resolved as her health bloomed. That's the power of taking time to select the right seeds to sow.

Please, don't skip this step, because you find it difficult. Self-analysis is never easy, but we can't expect change and transformation if we don't give it a good shot. Switch your attitude, believe in yourself, and get back to it. Remember: You cannot fail at this, you deserve this, and you will grow and learn from it—so don't you dare give up.

Congratulations! You have now selected your top three seeds of desire and the Whys that will allow them to grow. You are officially ready to sow your seeds.

SOWING YOUR INTENTION

What does it mean to "sow" in this context? It means planting your seeds of desire by setting a clear intention to surround those desires. In other words, it's time to put some skin in the game. To do this, we will create a simple ritual around setting your intentions/goals.

Let's have some creative fun sowing your seeds!

Optional Supplies:

- Your favorite music
- Essential oils and diffuser
- Candles
- Crystals

- Colored pencils/pens
- Feathers
- Leaves
- Flowers
- Scrapbooking supplies

PLANT YOUR SEEDS RITUAL

Find a quiet space where you can sit down, write, and draw.

Place some special objects around you—crystals, flowers, pictures of loved ones.

Put on your favorite soul-lifting music.

Light a candle.

Now, using the space below or the downloadable form provided at nourishmedicine.com/bloomresources, imagine planting your three seeds in the fertile soil of your expansive attitude/state of mind.

As you do so, plant your intentions by drawing or writing down your Seed Words using markers, your favorite pen, colored pencils, etc.

The purpose of this ritual is symbolic: to relax and have

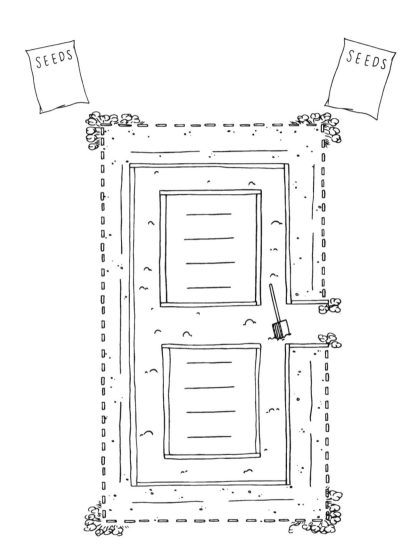

some fun while creating a tangible and beautiful space for your Seed Words. If you'd like to decorate the space below with stickers, dried flowers, other scrapbooking supplies, etc., go for it. If you're less inclined toward artwork, write them down in your best cursive with a nice pen. Just relax, and enjoy the process with an open mind and heart.

Once you have created a space for your seeds, I want you to imagine what your life will look like once those seeds have bloomed. Hold that image in your mind's eye.

Feel it.

Imagine it.

Relish it.

Congratulations! You have planted your seeds in a profound way, but you're not finished yet.

Since your seeds are still young and vulnerable, it is important they are remembered, nourished, and cared for every day throughout this process. Think about it, you can't throw seeds into fertile soil and expect them to grow without a significant level of care. You must water them, fertilize them, protect them from harsh weather, etc. Only then can you expect them to grow.

How do you do this with your seeds of desire?

- By watering them with optimism
- Nourishing them with an attitude of expansion
- Staying mindful of their presence

Studies have shown optimistic people and those with an open mind/attitude of expansion are more likely to expect positive outcomes. When people imagined—or pictured—a future where everything had turned out optimally for them, and did that for five minutes every day over a two-week period, their health and well-being improved.[1]

Here are some other ways you can care for your seeds by keeping them in the forefront of your mind.

FIND AN ACCOUNTABILITY BUDDY

Choose someone close to you who can help hold you accountable for your seeds. Tell a dear and trusted friend what you are doing and why and check in with them weekly. A quick text to let them know you are staying on track or experiencing roadblocks will go a long way.

JOIN THE LIFE IN BLOOM FACEBOOK GROUP TO CONNECT WITH FELLOW GARDENERS

Find a community of supportive like-minded women in the Life in Bloom Facebook Group. Your membership is included with the purchase of this book. See resources section for a link to join.

Daily Practice

It's important to reaffirm your intentions daily and connect with the energy and desire you have created in this process.

Here are a few ways to practice daily:

1. Visualization—when you first wake up in the morning, take a few moments to visualize your seeds in full, glorious bloom. Imagine what your life looks and feels like. It is important to create a strong mental image. In the short term, it will help you feel more optimistic. In the long term, staying focused on your goals and your desires will help you achieve them.
2. Meditation—meditate upon your intentions. Spend five to ten minutes focusing on breathing life into your desires or write about them in a journal. If you would like a guided meditation to help you, see the resources section at the end of this chapter for a link to a meditation you can download.
3. Use reminders—write your Seed Words and your Whys on sticky notes and place them around your home and office. Set

an alarm on your phone to be reminded of your intentions. You can also take a photo of your planted intentions paper and use it as a visual reminder on your desktop, phone, or tablet. This makes your journey a bit more private while giving you a consistent visual reminder.

As you sow, so shall you reap. Be deliberate about keeping a constant watchful eye on those seeds as we move forward.

THE PLIGHT OF PERFECTION

When you come upon a roadblock in this process, you must remember to be kind and compassionate with yourself. As modern women, we often struggle to find purpose and meaning amidst the chaos of our busy lives. Perhaps, our struggle would lessen if our ambitions weren't ensorcelled by the pursuit of perfection.

Perfection. It's an affliction that hinders our freedom and happiness to a terrible degree. Perfectionistic thinking, driven by a perfectionist attitude, can play a role in the development of eating disorders,[2] and increases our risk of anxiety and depression.[3] There is only one way to break this affliction: We must let go of the pursuit of perfection. Instead, we must accept—and dare I say celebrate—that nothing is going to be perfect or *stay* perfect, because life is not static.

Can the perfection-buck stop with our generation of women? I think it can, but we must be willing to practice compassion for ourselves first. Repeat after me: "I will focus on progress, not perfection. This is a process, not a race."

In addition to helping you make positive changes in your health, self-compassion has been shown to produce statistically and clinically significant reductions in depression, distress, as well as diabetes.[4]

That attitude of compassion—for yourself and others—contained within an expansive attitude, will allow you to find real, lasting healing for body, mind, and spirit.

With your seeds of desire and intention firmly planted in fertile soil, the next chapter will focus on how to nourish yourself—body, mind, and spirit—through specific nutrition, identifying food sensitivities, choosing the right supplements, and harnessing the little-known power of primary foods.

SOWING SEEDS

- You have permission to pursue your own well-being.
- Plant your garden seeds and think about how they will manifest in your life.
- Foster compassion for yourself.

Sowing Action Items:

1. Choose your seeds of desire from the Seed Word Box with care.

2. Next, whittle them down to your top three seeds using additional resources as needed.

3. Define your "Why" for each seed. What's your Why? Why are you taking this journey? What is it that you wish to achieve? What seeds do you wish to sow? Write them down and use additional resources as needed.

4. Switch your attitude to one of compassion for yourself; you'll need it to complete this journey and find real healing.

SOW Resources at nourishmedicine.com/bloomresources:

- Downloadable form to write your Top 3 Seed Words
- Guided Audio Meditation: Find Your Top 3 Seed Words
- Guided Audio Meditation: Find Your "Why"
- Access to Simon Sinek's Ted Talk on Finding your "Why"
- Downloadable form for Plant Your Seeds Ritual

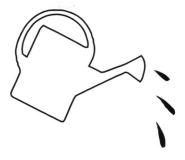

CHAPTER 3

Step 2: NOURISH— Love, Care, and Nourishment

———

In Step 1, we learned how to select your hardy seeds of desire and sow them with pure intention so they may manifest as you go through the Bloom process. In Step 2, we will learn how to create the ideal conditions for those seeds to grow and bloom using specific principles of physical, emotional, and spiritual nourishment.

To begin, we will start with everyone's favorite topic on nourishment: food.

FOOD AS INFORMATION

Food contains an enormous number of chemical substances, properly referred to as nutrients. Though most of us think about nutrients in terms of vitamins and minerals, there are, in fact, *thousands of nutrients*[1] that enter our bodies via the foods we eat every day, including amino acids, antioxidants, enzymes, essential fatty acids, fibers, prebiotics, probiotics, and others, in addition to essential vitamins and minerals.

To help paint a picture of how these nutrients interact with and nourish your body, picture a grand orchestra with nutrients as the musicians and you as the conductor. As conductors, we have the potential to feed a harmonious symphony by choosing foods that optimize our health, or create disharmony and cacophony by choosing foods that deplete our health.

In functional medicine, we view food as information, because what you eat sends your body powerful messages and cues. For example, nutrient interactions cause your immune system to respond to hormones, zap viruses and cancer cells, and to express—or not express—specific genes. When you think about it this way, it's hard to deny the simple act of eating as one of the most direct ways you can impact your health and longevity.

In other words, food may very well be the most powerful medicine on the planet.

However, nutrient interactions aren't the only way food impacts health. There is also the mental and emotional impacts food—or the *promise* of food—has on our physiology. You probably learned about the most famous example of this in elementary school science class: Pavlov's dog. Based on his studies, Nobel-prize winning scientist Ivan Pavlov, coined the term "psychic secretions,"[2] which we now refer to as "the cephalic response of food" or "anticipatory physiological regulation."

What does this mean? When you anticipate, sense, smell, and/or think about food, it causes your body to begin the digestion process by producing saliva, before the food has even graced your lips. One of the most interesting parts of this whole process, in relation to the mental and emotional impacts of food, is that the cephalic response is driven by the vagus nerve—the largest nerve in the body, which connects your brain to the gut.[3]

With this understanding, you can see why it is so important to slow down enough to really *think* about your food; to perceive, appreciate, and sense it fully, thereby activating that initial phase of digestion. In contrast, if you feel stressed out, distracted, or are eating on the go, your entire digestive process will be compromised from the start.

Beyond just slowing down, studies have shown positive or negative thoughts can affect digestion and nutrient processing (think about trying to eat and digest your food when you're upset versus happy), and that is likely related to the gut-brain connection via the vagus nerve.[4] Likewise, our interactions and attitudes toward food can have a distinct impact on our spirits. A perfect example is food shared at the dinner table. Numerous studies—coupled with good old-fashioned common sense—demonstrate families who consistently sit down together at the dinner table are more bonded, and children who sit with their parents to eat have better life and health outcomes across the board.[5,6]

So, is it the food or the company profoundly nourishing our spirit? It's both. You can't have good health without good nutrition, and as new research is proving, you can't have good health without regular, loving, social connection either.[7]

As discussed in the beginning of this chapter, nutrients are only one part of the nourishment puzzle. Combine good food with mindfulness in a social setting and you've got a perfect recipe for healing and nourishing your body, mind, and spirit.

Michael Pollan, *New York Times* best-selling author and expert on science and food, speaks at length in his books and publications, such as *The Omnivore's Dilemma*, about how the Western diet has radically shifted from whole foods to refined foods made up of simple carbs.[8] When and why did this happen? After World War II, processed food made its way from the battlefields into the North American kitchen. With food companies' success in providing inexpensive, processed food to our troops and more women working outside the home, the country was eager to embrace the new concept of "convenience foods."

However, as things got more "convenient," we lost sight of the value in traditional cooking methods that had sustained us since time immemorial. In essence, we forgot how to cook. The Baby Boomer generation shunned the Depression-era generation who still had this culinary wisdom. Unfortunately, as we lose our elders, we lose their time-honored nutritional cooking methods. Traditional cooking methods were developed for survival and economy while often enhancing foods' nutritional value and aiding digestion and immunity.

One of my favorite traditional foods (which is experiencing a revival) is bone broth. Bone broths were born out of necessity to avoid wasting food while creating a nutritious base for soups, sauces, and stews. As the bones are simmered with water and vegetables, the process extracts amino acids, gelatin, glycines, and glycosaminoglycans, which are all very healing and beneficial for your gut, your body's mucosa, your eyeballs, and all your collagenous structures, including your nails, teeth, and bones.[9,10] These days, traditional bone broth is often replaced by the bouillon cube or quick-made commercial stock, which gives you the flavor of broth but lacks in nutrients.

Fermenting foods, such as vegetables, dairy, and beans, is also a lost art in many ways. The fermentation, pickling, or souring process naturally preserves food while creating a plethora of probiotics that nourish your gut and enhance immunity.[11] While many of us may make it a point to consume yogurt or other pickled products regularly, too often, those yogurts are loaded with sugar and artificial ingredients, and commercial pickles aren't traditionally fermented pickles, they are made using added vinegar, which means you're not getting the probiotic benefit of a traditionally pickled food.

In traditional Mexican cuisine, all corn-based foods were prepared using a nearly forgotten process called nixtamalization, in which the freshly ground corn was mixed with lime or ashes. Adding those elements extracts the B vitamins, makes more calcium and protein available, and reduces citric acid—an anti-nutrient that blocks the absorption of calcium and other minerals.[12] Needless to say, nixtamalization is not used in modern production of corn products.

Another nearly lost culinary art is the simple act of soaking or sprouting cereals, grains, and legumes to reduce phytates (another anti-nutrient that inhibits nutrient absorption) while improving bioavailability of zinc and vitamin C.[13]

THE HEALTHIER SIDE OF BREAD

Whether bread is healthy is the subject of great debate among the nutritional and integrative functional medicine community. Though many people with sensitivities to wheat, gluten, and other grains would be well-advised to avoid bread, the issue with bread may lie in the loss of its traditional preparation.

Up until the twentieth century, bread was made by incubating flour and water with natural fermented yeast or a sourdough starter for an entire day. During that time, the natural yeasts and cultures would break down much of the gluten while neutralizing anti-nutrients and creating probiotics. Hence, many nutritional experts believe the problem with bread and gluten may have more to do with its modern fast-rise preparation and the intense hybridization of modern wheat, than the bread itself.

Yes, you can buy sourdough at the supermarket, but if you look closely, most inexpensive sourdoughs are made with conventional wheat and commercial yeast, and not allowed to ferment twenty-four hours as a traditional sourdough would.

The effect of diet on future generations has been studied at length by famous physicians and researchers like Weston A.

Price, a dentist who spent years studying the health and bone structures of indigenous cultures. His discoveries, made famous by the book *Nourishing Traditions* and the Weston A. Price Foundation, confirmed processed foods cause a notable decline in the dental and overall health of future generations.[14] Likewise, Francis Pottenger, a medical doctor famous for his work: *Pottenger's Cats: A Study in Nutrition,* proved how replacing a cat's natural diet of raw foods with cooked foods degraded their physical and mental health with each generation.[15] Pottenger believed that the same effects took place in humans who had turned away from their natural and ancestral diets, and those genetic weaknesses could be reversed by returning to an unprocessed diet.

It is my belief that the current rise in gut-health issues, digestive complaints, nutrient deficiencies, food sensitivities, and chronic inflammatory disease is largely due to the abandonment of our traditional culinary framework compounded by an increased toxic load. Despite the gains we have experienced since World War II in freedom, technology, and equal rights, the loss of those simple cooking skills, along with our more sedate way of life, has been detrimental to us all.

WHAT HUNTER GATHERERS CAN TEACH US ABOUT WORK-LIFE BALANCE

According to a book on Stone Age economics,[16] in hunter-gatherer communities, women would spend one day gathering enough food to feed their families for three days. Then, the rest of their time was spent on leisure activities, such as embroidery or visiting with friends from other camps. For each day spent at home, the women would spend only about three hours on housework (cracking nuts, fetching water and firewood, etc.), and take the rest of the day "off." They maintained that balanced routine of work and leisure throughout the year.

For a long stretch of human development, we devoted only one to three hours to hard work a day, and even then, we spent a lot of time visiting with people and pursuing useful hobbies. We weren't and aren't meant to be on our own and on the go all the time.

AVA'S STORY

When she came to me, Ava had horrible irritable bowel syndrome, along with stomach pain and rashes all over her body. I did my typical work up, which showed that, ultimately, she needed to nourish herself better by changing her diet. But there was a snag: She had already planned a mission trip to Thailand. She was going to be there for a month and wouldn't have any option as to what she could or couldn't eat.

Fortunately, Thai cuisine is very traditional, even today. To her surprise, her irritable bowel syndrome completely reversed during her trip, purely by virtue of eating foods prepared in a traditional manner.

FOOD SENSITIVITIES

When I talk about food sensitivities, I'm not talking about

an allergic reaction to food, which is known as an IgE-mediated response. A food allergy will cause symptoms like swollen lips or hives. A food sensitivity, on the other hand, is a delayed hypersensitivity response, which is triggered by IgG antibodies—food antigen and antibody complexes to which the immune system reacts.[17]

Food sensitivities occur because of leaky gut syndrome, also known as hyper-permeability of the intestinal wall.[18] I see food sensitivities due to leaky gut in my practice all the time and treating them does not have to be difficult. But before we get into treatment protocols, let's learn a little more about leaky gut, and why it afflicts so many otherwise healthy people.

Your gastrointestinal tract is a long tube that runs from the mouth all the way to the anus, and includes all the organs that contribute to digestion and waste removal, such as your esophagus, stomach, and intestinal tract. Once a food, substance, or toxin enters our body and reaches the gut, it must then get by the "guardian at the gate," known as the gastric epithelium. Its job is to protect and discern what foods, nutrients, chemicals, etc., are safe to be absorbed into our body.

Now, picture your intestines as an absorbent yet tightly woven net. This net serves as a physical and functional filter between our inner body and the outside environment, allowing tiny, easy-to-absorb nutrients to flow in, while larger harmful substances and pathogens are kept out and eliminated through the bowels. When the intestinal wall becomes compromised due to toxins from food,[19] medications such as NSAIDS,[20] stress, gut flora imbalance,[21] and chemicals,[22] the tightly knit holes in your net become weak, stretched, and can easily tear.

These tiny tears leave the compromised gut wide open to undigested food proteins, which cause an immune system response. Sensing these "foreign invaders," the immune system goes into an inflammatory attack mode to reject these unwanted substances. Symptoms of this "red alert" I have observed in practice and research may include congestion, diarrhea, a rash, bloating, brain fog, joint ache, depression,[23] and—you guessed it—food sensitivities.[17]

When a patient comes to me with symptoms of leaky gut and food sensitivities, two things I suggest are a simple elimination diet (the gold standard in functional medicine) and an IgG food sensitivity test. Elimination diets have not only been shown to help resolve gut-related health issues like IBS,[24] but they also help us identify causal factors and trigger foods.[25]

TOP EIGHT SYMPTOMS OF FOOD SENSITIVITY

- Anxiety
- Brain fog
- Bloating
- Chronic congestion
- Fatigue
- Joint aches
- Headache
- Rashes

Complex health problems often require simple solutions. It doesn't get simpler than removing a few things from your daily diet to replace with more nourishing foods. Remember, food is information; therefore, I recommend anyone reading this book, regardless of whether you have digestive issues, to take the time to eliminate the following most common reactionary foods for four weeks. After four weeks, reintroduce them slowly, one at time every three days, so you can observe your body's reaction and pinpoint the exact issue.

The most common reactionary or "inflammatory" foods to eliminate from your diet:

- Gluten
- Dairy

- Grains (including corn)
- Beans
- Soy
- Eggs
- Sugar
- Alcoholic beverages

Now, before you have a melt-down at the thought of eliminating bread and cheese, remember your seeds and your big Why, check the status of your attitude (this is an opportunity for growth and expansion), and consider all the amazing new foods you can eat and experiment with such as:

- Gluten-free, grain-free breads, chips, and tortillas.
- Dairy-free creamers, milks, and cheeses.
- Replace grains, beans, and legumes with more vegetables, sweet potatoes, veggie noodles, soy-free shirataki noodles, riced cauliflower, coconut, and almond flour.
- Replace soy-based products with coconut and nut-based products like coconut and almond milk.
- To replace eggs in baking, mix one tablespoon of flax meal with one tablespoon of water. Soak until it gels and use 1:1 in place of eggs.
- Sweeteners such as natural stevia, raw honey, coconut sugar, and xylitol.
- Kombucha in place of alcohol—you will be surprised how

it relaxes you and calms the mind (especially when enjoyed from a wine glass).

I also recommend reviewing "Dr. Alex's Elimination Diet Quick Start Guide" at the end of this chapter, which includes sample recipes and menu plans and downloading a version of the guide and menu plan at nourishmedicine. com/bloomresources.

Just in case that's not enough to get you motivated, consider the common beneficial side effects of an elimination diet:

- Weight loss
- Tons more energy
- Clearer, more youthful skin
- Better sleep
- Improved digestion and elimination
- Reduced cravings for sugar and other processed foods
- Laser-sharp focus and concentration
- Easier periods
- More balanced hormones
- A higher sex drive
- Stable mood and increased feeling of happiness and well-being
- Better endurance
- Fewer aches and pains
- Fewer headaches

- Better vision
- Improved memory
- A greater awareness of your body and what "healthy" feels like
- Less worry knowing you are giving your body what it needs to heal

As you go through this process of nourishment, keep your end-goal in mind, remember your Seeds Words, and join us in the Life in Bloom Facebook group for support. You've got this—now get to it!

TEN GUIDING PRINCIPLES TO EVERYDAY EATING FOR VIBRANT HEALTH

1. Eat Real Food

Food is information; therefore, we want to provide our bodies with the right information to heal, rebuild, and thrive. The three best ways to "eat real food" are:

1. Purge your diet of processed foods (even the "all natural" varieties) such as: fast food, artificial sweeteners, frozen dinners, packaged foods, canned foods, boxed foods, sodas, and cold cuts.
2. Stick to the perimeter of the grocery store and avoid the middle aisles where the packaged and processed foods live. Try to buy fresh meat and vegetables, and don't eat anything out of a box if you can help it.

3. Shop your local farmer's market to get fresh food that's super-nutritious and naturally grown.

2. Eat a Rainbow of Fruits and Vegetables

Fruits and vegetables contain a huge number of essential chemical substances and phytonutrients (the chemicals that give fruits and vegetables their color and flavor). All these different substances work together to support health in numerous ways—from cancer prevention[26,27,28] to heart health.[29,30,31]

The more colorful your diet, the better—and leafy green vegetables are king. Aim to make half your daily vegetable intake green and the rest colorful.

How many servings of fruits and veggies should you eat daily? I suggest aiming for ten to seventeen servings of vegetables daily, and no more than two to three servings of fruit. A serving is defined as one cup of raw leafy greens or half of all other vegetables, one medium fruit the size of a baseball or half a cup of chopped or cooked fruit.

Why do I recommend so many fruits and vegetables when the USDA recommends less? Because our bodies require more nutrients, antioxidants, etc. to repair, heal, and functional optimally in this less-than-perfect modern world. Remember, this isn't your grandmother's dinner.

Now, if you're thinking, "How the heck am I going to eat that much produce every day?" Let me assure you, it's a lot easier than you may think. Here are the tips I share with my patients on getting their ten to seventeen servings per day:

- Start slow—if you're eating less than the recommendation above, start by adding in one extra serving of fruit or veggies every three days. Replace your usual snack with a piece of fruit one day, then add a cup (or two) of veggie-based soup to your lunch the next day. Before you know it, you'll have worked your way up to ten to seventeen veggies and two to three fruits.
- Explore—different global cuisines, nutrition philosophies, and their vegetable dishes. For example, raw food and vegetarian cookbooks have a lot of creative ways to enjoy veggies in dips, sauces, as snacks, etc.
- Get creative—by incorporating vegetable soups, salads, steamed vegetables, raw fruits, vegetables as snacks, vegetable drinks, green juices, etc.

Here's what a typical day of ten to seventeen veggies and two to three fruits looks like:

- Breakfast: A green protein smoothie with one fruit, one to

two cups of greens such as spinach, kale, or collards, and half of an avocado (three servings veggies, one fruit)
- Snack: An apple with almond butter (one fruit)
- Lunch: A big salad with two to three cups lettuce, cucumber, carrots, a protein, and pumpkin seeds. (two to four servings of veggies)
- Snack: Guacamole with carrots and celery and a pickle (two to three servings veggies)
- Dinner: Seven-veggie meat sauce with spiralized veggie, gluten-free, or shirataki noodles (four to six servings of vegetables)

Total for the day: two fruits, ten to sixteen veggies. Easy, right? You just have to think a little differently, and visit my website for recipes and tips on eating the rainbow in the resources section.

3. Eat Healthy Fats

This is a loaded topic. Of all the food and nutrition controversies out there, fats dominate the confusion. Just last year, after decades of low-fat-is-heart-healthy dogma, *The New York Times* ran an expose titled: "How the Sugar Industry Shifted Blame to Fat"[32] on how Harvard scientists were paid off by the sugar industry in the 1950s to point the blame of heart disease on fat, when sugar had been the real culprit all along. That's a game-changer.

Yet those of us who grew up in the seventies and eighties have been conditioned to fear fat (especially saturated fats). We have a hard time accepting its role in health and healing. So, here are the real facts on fat:

Omega-3 fats, found in fatty fish, flax seeds, chia seeds, and walnuts are associated with anti-inflammatory benefits across the board.[33] You want these fats in your diet every day.

In contrast, omega-6 fats from vegetable oils and other common cooking oils are very inflammatory.[34] You need to limit these fats for two reasons.

1. They are everywhere, so it's easy to get too much of them. In fact, most of us consume a ratio of 20:1 omega 6 to omega 3, when 2:1 would be ideal.
2. No one living in the twenty-first century needs more inflammation in their body, period.

Your best sources of beneficial fats include:

- Avocado oil
- Coconut oil
- Extra Virgin Olive Oil
- Ghee or clarified butter (preferably from pasture-raised cows and not during the elimination diet)
- Wild salmon and other cold water, low-mercury fish

- Avocados
- Walnuts, hemp seeds, chia seeds, flax seeds and super-fresh flaxseed oil
- High-quality, pasture-raised animal fats such as butter, lard, and tallow

Saturated fats have been vilified for the last fifty years as the leading cause of heart disease. However, new research is showing saturated fats do not cause heart disease[35] and is instead pointing the blame at sugar and processed carbohydrates.[36] Based on this new research, the study of health-promoting traditional diets, and my own clinical experience, I do recommend including moderate amounts of high-quality saturated fats in your diet. When it comes to animal-based fats choose butter, lard, and tallow from healthy animals raised on pasture. This gives them a superior fatty acid profile and flavor. If you're sensitive to dairy, skip the butter or opt for clarified butter or ghee, which have had their milk solids removed.

For vegetable-based saturated fats, you can't go wrong with coconut oil. It's best to choose virgin, but for those who don't like the flavor of coconut, refined coconut oil is okay. Palm kernel oil is healthful as well, but is generally not a sustainably sourced product, which is why I recommend coconut, first and foremost.

4. Eat Protein at Every Meal

Protein is found everywhere in the body and helps build muscle, repair tissues, regulate metabolism, and power enzymatic reactions throughout organs and systems. Given the vast role protein plays in our bodies, we need to replenish our stores regularly.

Here are some tips on choosing high-quality proteins from animal and plant-based sources:

- For meats and poultry—choose grass-fed/pasture-raised and organic whenever possible. Pasture-raised/grass-fed meats like beef, for example, are higher in anti-inflammatory fats and much healthier for you.[37] Organic meats from animals raised on organic feed and/or grass are a better option than conventional, but pasture-raised and/or grass-fed meats are superior and are typically available at farmer's markets, natural foods stores, food co-ops, local butchers, and many grocery stores. See resources section for more information on finding a local source.
- For fish and seafood—look for wild-caught, sustainably harvested fish and seafood with low-mercury content and avoid farm raised. This typically means choosing smaller fish, such as wild-caught salmon, sardines, anchovies, and shrimp. See resources section for a link to the Environmental Working Group's guide on choosing healthful fish from clean waters.
- For plant-based proteins—avoid soy products, unless they

are organic and fermented or cultured—such as tempeh, miso, or tamari. The reason is soybeans are highly allergenic and loaded with anti-nutrients and phytoestrogens,[38] which is typically bad news for anyone with autoimmune, gut, or hormonal issues. Fermented soy products, however, are a better choice as the fermentation process neutralizes those anti-nutrients.[39] Beans and other legumes may be fine post-elimination diet for those who can tolerate them, as are nuts and seeds and hemp or pea protein powders. Please steer clear of soy protein and soy protein powders, period. These products are highly processed and very hard to digest.

To determine how much protein you need, take your body's weight in pounds, divide it by 0.75, and the resulting number is how many grams of protein you (as a woman) should be eating per day. If this seems like too much at once, start by consuming a palm-sized amount of protein with every meal.

DR. ALEX'S TOP PICKS FOR PROTEIN POWDERS

Protein powders are a convenient way to get more protein in your diet and can be a great addition to smoothies and green drinks. However, not all protein powders are created equal in terms of nutrition—in fact, with their long lists of synthetic, processed ingredients, many of them are just plain junk food.

Here are my top favorite protein powders that provide the purest, cleanest source of protein and are allowed on the elimination diet:

1. Organic pea protein isolate—an excellent plant-based vegan option made from yellow split peas.

2. Organic hemp protein—another highly nutritious plant-based vegan protein powder with a balanced fatty acid profile.

3. Hydrolyzed grass-fed beef protein powder—an excellent source of protein and has many of the healing properties of bone broth.

4. Hydrolyzed grass-fed collagen—similar properties to the beef protein powder and is a staple for helping maintain youthful skin, hair, and nails. It is tasteless and can be added to any beverage for a quick protein boost.

You will find specific brand recommendations and links to these protein powders at nourishmedicine.com/bloomresources, plus a green drink/ protein shake tutorial coming up later in the chapter.

5. Eat a Variety of Foods

Though we are all creatures of habit, it is essential we not default to eating the same foods every day—even healthy foods—for a couple of reasons:

1. It limits the amount and types of nutrients you're receiving.

2. When you eat the same foods day in and day out, it increases the chances your immune system will "see" and react to the food, which can lead to food sensitivities.

You can take this a step further by eating in-season for superior nutrition and health benefits. Eating in-season not only ensures year-round variety in your diet, but it can also help ward off seasonal ailments. For example, many indigenous cultures consumed nettles and/or dandelion greens in the spring, which help cleanse the liver and reduce the likelihood of seasonal allergies.[40]

6. Support Healthy Blood Sugar

The amount of starch and sugar consumed in the modern diet, coupled with our sedentary lifestyles, leads to blood sugar crashes and energy dips.

Studies have shown that eating less sugar and starchy carbs is beneficial for blood sugar and decreases your risk of diabetes, low-immunity, and heart disease.[41] To cut carbs without feeling deprived, replace them with vegetables or healthy fats at snack time, decrease the amount of sugar you consume daily to twenty-five grams or less (less is much better), and make sure no more than one-eighth to one-quarter of your plate is made up of starchy vegetables, bread, or grains.

7. Do a Thirty-Day Elimination Diet

See above and "Dr. Alex's Elimination Diet Quick Start Guide" at the end of this chapter for detailed information on how and why to do this. Get to it!

8. Stay Hydrated

If you're not hydrating regularly, it can make you feel very tired. Dehydration causes a drop in blood volume, which makes your heart work harder to deliver oxygen to your muscles and skin. Studies have shown even mild dehydration of just 2 percent can cause people to feel unfocused, fatigued, and anxious.[42]

How much water do you need? I recommend six to eight glasses of water every day, while avoiding fruit juice, black teas, energy drinks, and soda. Carrying a glass or stainless steel water bottle with you will make this a no-brainer. If you don't like water, try infusing it with whole slices of fruit, such as lemon, berries, or orange, or opt for sparkling water, green tea, or herbal tea.

9. Eat Traditional Superfoods

Such as the bone broths, fermented foods, soaked nuts and seeds, and others mentioned in the "Not Your Grandmother's Dinner" section of this chapter.

10. Eat with Joy

Have you ever heard the saying, "Drinking beer with lots of cheer is better than eating bread with lots of dread"? Food, community, and connection are so important. Gathering socially and joyfully with your friends and loved ones for food brings a different kind of information to your system. It is important to eat happily, mindfully, and gratefully, and to enjoy the experience—no matter what you're eating.

SOPHIE'S STORY

Sophie came to see me for a nutritional therapy approach for her new diagnosis of rheumatoid arthritis. When I first talked to her about the elimination diet and the ten steps to eating for everyday vibrant health, she became very angry. She kept asking, "How can I not eat pizza? How can I not eat pasta? How can I not eat that? That's going to be tough. How can I participate in life and community, if I don't eat these foods?"

Eventually, after much discussion, she agreed to follow a custom elimination diet that also included restrictions on nuts, caffeine, and all cheeses—three foods that tend to be troublesome in those with autoimmune conditions.

Despite her initial reaction, she followed through. Within about a month, her pain went away. Her arthritis has not progressed, and she has maintained pain-free joints by eating in a nourishing way and eliminating her trigger foods that we discovered through the elimination diet and food sensitivity testing: nightshade vegetables (tomatoes, potatoes, eggplant, and peppers), gluten, dairy, and eggs. By sticking to this program, she is living a fuller life than she would have otherwise. That's the power of nourishment.

NOURISHING THE SOUL WITH PRIMARY FOOD

Several years ago, The Institute of Integrative Nutrition created a concept known as "primary food"—but the name is a bit misleading as it's not food-related. Our "primary foods" are the things—people, activities, spiritual practices, hobbies, traditions, places, laughter, prayer, etc.—that bring us nourishment on a spiritual level.

Primary foods feed the soul, and when you nourish yourself this way, your body rewards you by releasing a slew of feel-good hormones and chemicals that serve much in the same way food does.

If you have forgotten what it means to feed your soul in this way, start by thinking about what brings you pleasure and joy, and ask yourself these questions:

- What did you love to do as a child?
- What did you love to do as a teenager?
- What did you enjoy doing before you got so darn busy keeping up with your own life?

This should stir up some memories like, "I used to love playing outside," or, "I'd always enjoy taking a long walk after work with a girlfriend," or, "I used to unwind by playing the guitar."

DISCOVERING YOUR "PRIMARY FOODS"

Ask yourself:

- "What did I love to do as a child?"
- "What do I love to do for fun?"
- "What's something I've always wanted to do and never tried?"
- "What was the last thing I did that made me feel accomplished?"
- "What was the last activity I engaged in that made me feel alive?"

Once we enter the grown-up world, it can feel as though all our resources go to advancing our career, running our family, or taking care of others, instead of doing the things that nourish our soul. Though we may long to go meet up with friends for coffee or try out for the local theater, finding the time and space to organize your hobbies can feel daunting, indulgent, or worse, non-productive (gasp!).

Well, let me ask you this: Would you consider eating a healthy meal as something indulgent and a waste of time? No, of course not, because if you don't eat, you'll get sick, tired, and cranky. Same goes with consuming enough "primary foods;" if you don't nourish your soul on a regular basis you are going to get sick, tired, cranky, and, ultimately, burnt out.

Have you ever wondered why so many smart, successful, loving women are so desperately unhappy beneath the surface? Not to oversimplify the pursuit of happiness or negate the real issues often surrounding depression, I would bet, at the very least, they are suffering from a serious case of soul-starvation brought on by a lack of primary foods.

Personally, my primary foods are gardening, reading, and playing the cello—something I enjoyed doing as a child and have picked back up again. Gardening, on the other hand, was something I had always wanted to do, but never made the time and space for it. When I finally started a garden two years ago, I did it with my family, and it's been such a blessing for all of us—and the inspiration for this book. This brings up an important point: Nourishing yourself this way doesn't have to be an isolated experience unless that's what you desire. These things must be done in "real life," so why not include your children, husband, partner, friends, pets, etc.? The point is to make time to nourish your spirit every day.

You have taken a tremendous step in this process by learning to nourish yourself through honoring your individual nutritional needs. Though changing your relationship to food can be a challenge, you have set yourself up for success by taking the time to identify and plant those seeds of desire and holding true to that attitude of expansion and growth. I encourage you to check out the Step 2 resources—including some of my favorite elimination diet recipes on the Bloom website—and to connect with others following this process in the Life in Bloom Facebook group.

Our journey continues in the next chapter with Step 3, where you will learn how to get grounded and build physical, mental, and emotional strength using proven restorative practices.

Remember, the grass is greener where you water it, so take care to consistently and deliberately nourish your seeds.

NOURISHING YOUR WHOLE SELF

- What type of cuisine did your grandparents eat? Do you have a specific cuisine of your family's origin? What can you do to incorporate some of those (or others mentioned) traditional cooking methods into your life?

- Do any of the symptoms of food sensitivities or leaky gut syndrome sound familiar to you? What steps in the "Ten Steps to Eating for Vibrant Health" do you need to incorporate in your nourishment routine?

- What nourishes your spirit that you're not doing? What can you do to fix that?

Nourishing Action Items:

1. Plan to start your elimination diet using the list provided above OR come over to nourishmedicine.com/bloomresources for my Elimination Diet Quick Start Guide and recipe downloads.

2. Print out the Ten Steps to Vibrant Everyday Eating Guide from nourishmedicine.com/bloomresources and tape it on your fridge. Implement those steps into your daily routine.

3. Seek out your primary foods: the hobbies, activities, and things that will nourish your spirit and soul.

4. If you're struggling with the elimination diet or implementing the Ten Guiding Principles to Vibrant Eating, check out the resource section below and hop on the Life in Bloom Facebook group for support.

NOURISH Resources at nourishmedicine.com/bloomresources:

- Green Smoothie Guide
- Dr. Alex's Elimination Diet Quick Start Guide
- Recipe Guidebook
- Ten Steps to Vibrant Eating Guide
- Additional online recipe resources
- Recommendations for discount and specialty natural foods resources

Your Intention/Goal: Eliminate the following most common reactionary foods for four weeks and replace them with non-reactive foods to nourish your body.

Your Why: You are eliminating these reactionary foods so that you can discover what food sensitivities you may have and which foods your body thrives on.

Reactionary Foods to Eliminate for Four Weeks:

- Gluten—found in breads, some grains, flours, sauces, and processed foods
- Dairy
- Grains—including corn, rice, couscous, pastas, quinoa, millet, wheat, spelt, teff, rye, barley, etc.
- Beans and Legumes—includes peanuts as a legume
- Soy—beans, milk, yogurt, tofu, oil, edamame, soy sauce, etc. Read labels carefully as soy is in many packaged foods as an oil or soy lecithin.
- Eggs
- Sugar—white sugar, corn syrup, high fructose corn syrup, sucanat, turbinado, cane sugar, sugar in the raw
- Alcoholic beverages

Foods You CAN Eat During the Four-Week Elimination Diet:

- Vegetables—all kinds including potatoes, sweet potatoes, and plantains. Aim for thirteen-seventeen servings a day
- Fruits—up to two servings per day
- Meats and poultry—preferably pasture-raised/grass-fed and/or organic. Wild game is also an excellent source
- Wild-caught fish and seafood
- Grain-free flours—for baking, thickening, dredging, and "breading" such as coconut flour, almond flour, and tapioca flour
- Vegetable and seaweed crisps and chips—provided they are not cooked in inflammatory oils (choose coconut oil, olive oil, and avocado oil)
- Healthy fats—olive oil, coconut oil, and avocado oil
- Nuts and seeds—except peanuts, which are a legume
- Sugar-free, peanut-free nut butters—such as almond butter, tahini, and sunflower butter
- Sugar substitutes—such as stevia and xylitol. Coconut sugar and raw honey are allowed in very limited quantities
- To drink—plenty of filtered water, kombucha, coffee (one cup a day without dairy or refined sugar, please), herbal, and green teas

HOW TO START RE-INTRODUCING REACTIONARY FOODS AFTER FOUR WEEKS

Patience is a virtue when it comes to the re-introduction phase. If you reintroduce those reactionary foods too quickly, you will wind up missing crucial information and possibly negating this whole process.

- Start re-introducing the eliminated foods one at a time
- Observe how you feel for three days before introducing another
- Write down your observations

Signs of Food Sensitivities to Look for When Re-Introducing Eliminated/Reactionary Foods

- Acne
- An unwanted change in mood
- Athlete's foot or other fungal issues
- Bad breath
- Brain fog
- Canker sores
- Congestion
- Constipation
- Diarrhea
- Digestive upset
- Dry eyes
- Fatigue

- Gas and/or bloating
- Headaches
- Insomnia
- Itching or skin irritation
- Joint pain
- Puffy face or eyes
- Rashes, irritation, or redness that may occur anywhere on your skin, including around your anus or genitals
- Scratchy throat
- Stomachache
- Weight gain

7-DAY SAMPLE ELIMINATION DIET MENU PLAN

The following is a sample of how one week on the elimination diet would look. Some featured recipes are listed at the back of this section; others can be found at nourishmedicine.com/bloomresources.

You can access dozens of delicious BLOOM-friendly recipes on my website, or you can design your own menu plan and recipes sticking within the non-reactive food limits.

Day 1:

- Breakfast: *Nut Butter Pie Smoothie* and a cup of coffee or green tea

- Morning Snack: An apple with almond butter
- Lunch: *Green Goddess Cobb Salad* with a cup of *Bone Broth* or *Easy Chicken Broth*
- Afternoon Snack: Crudité with baba ganoush or your favorite soy-free, dairy-free dressing or dairy-free pesto
- Dinner: *Buffalo Burger in a Napa Wrap*
- Drink at least eight glasses of water

Day 2:

- Breakfast: *Sweet Potato Breakfast Hash* and a cup of coffee or green tea
- Morning Snack: *Green Drink/Smoothie*
- Lunch: *Steak Salad with Mojo Dressing* or a vegetable-based soup with shrimp or chicken
- Afternoon Snack: A cup (or more) of bone broth with carrot sticks
- Dinner: *Phenomenal Pho* (recipe available on my website)
- Drink at least eight glasses of water

Day 3:

- Breakfast: *Cinnamon Chai Protein Smoothie* and a cup of coffee or green tea
- Morning Snack: *Goji Chocolate Nut Bar*
- Lunch: Leftover *Phenomenal Pho*

- Afternoon Snack: Raw veggies with *Pumped Up Guacamole with Watercress and Pomegranate Arils*
- Dinner: Chicken or turkey stew with potatoes and loads of veggies, OR grilled chicken or turkey strips (marinated in your favorite sugar-free, soy-free marinade or dressing) with baked potato and salad
- Drink at least eight glasses of water

Day 4:

- Breakfast: *Pumpkin Pie Smoothie* and a cup of coffee or green tea
- Morning Snack: Diced avocado and mango fruit salad with hemp seeds (chop up ½ an avocado and one mango, add hemp seeds and a squirt of lime juice and enjoy)
- Lunch: Leftovers from the night before (stew or grilled chicken or turkey) with a cup of *Bone Broth* or *Easy Chicken Broth* OR *Watercress Almond Soup with Chicken or Shrimp*
- Afternoon Snack: *Green Drink/Smoothie*
- Dinner: *Grilled Salmon with Pineapple Salsa* and grilled vegetables of choice (make enough salmon and grilled vegetables to save some for the next day)
- Drink at least eight glasses of water

Day 5:

- Breakfast: Veggie and meat scramble with 2-3 strips of bacon

with greens and leftover grilled vegetables and a cup of coffee or green tea
- Morning Snack: Celery sticks stuffed with nut butter
- Lunch: Leftover *Grilled Salmon* with lemon or lime and grilled vegetables with a cup of *Bone Broth* or *Easy Chicken Broth*
- Afternoon Snack: *Double Dark Chocolate Smoothie*
- Dinner: Spiralized veggie noodles with lamb, bison, or turkey-based meat sauce
- Drink at least eight glasses of water

Day 6:

- Breakfast: *Chillin Cucumber Smoothie* and a cup of coffee or green tea
- Morning Snack: *Goji Chocolate Nut Bar*
- Lunch: *Steak Salad with Mojo Dressing* OR *Herby Chilled Beet Soup with Avocado*
- Afternoon Snack: Nori rolls stuffed with shredded veggies, pickled ginger, and avocado
- Dinner: Roasted organic/free-range chicken with sweet potatoes and a variety of roasted vegetables such as zucchini, leeks, carrots, etc. Make enough sweet potatoes and veggies for leftovers
- Drink at least eight glasses of water

Day 7:

- Breakfast: Green Drink/Smoothie and a cup of coffee or green tea
- Morning Snack: Diced fresh pineapple cubes with crushed macadamia nuts
- Lunch: Leftover roasted chicken and veggies
- Afternoon Snack: Guacamole with chopped veggies
- Dinner: *Ground Beef Picadillo* with Lettuce Cups
- Drink at least eight glasses of water

ELIMINATION-DIET-FRIENDLY RECIPE SAMPLES

(more available at: nourishmedicine.com/bloomresources)

Breakfast Recipes

Sweet Potato Breakfast Hash

This savory-sweet hash makes a hearty, nutrient-dense breakfast that will leave you feeling full and satisfied for hours. For easy morning prep, you can roast the potatoes the night before, then just add bacon or premade, organic, nitrate-free sausage and wilt in some greens.

Serves 2

Ingredients:

- 1 medium sweet potato, roasted
- 2 green onions, sliced
- 3 strips of nitrate-free, preferably organic bacon OR 2 nitrate-free, sugar-free, preferably organic sausages
- 2 teaspoons extra virgin olive oil or coconut oil
- Handful of fresh spinach
- 2 tablespoons salsa or red or green mojo (mojo recipes listed below)

Procedure:

1. Cook bacon or sausage according to directions. Remove from pan and set aside.
2. In the same pan, add pre-baked sweet potato with skin on (lots of nutrients in there) and mash up.
3. Add spinach to the same skillet and wilt in with sweet potato.
4. Add back the bacon or sausage and heat through.
5. Top with your favorite salsa or mojo and enjoy.

Drink and Smoothie Recipes

Nut Butter Pie Smoothie

Nut fans will nod their heads in approval upon first sip of this creamy treat. It may seem too good to be labeled a healthy breakfast, but this smoothie offers a good dose of minerals and antioxidants from nuts and spices. Dial up the flavor with cinnamon (great for controlling blood sugar) and nutmeg (potent antibacterial).

Serves 2

Ingredients:

- 1¼ cups cold tea such black or green tea
- ¼ cup coconut milk
- 3 tablespoons nut butter, such as almond or cashew
- 2 tablespoons chia seeds
- 1 scoop vanilla or chocolate protein powder (choose pea, hemp, hydrolyzed beef, or hydrolyzed collagen)
- ¼ teaspoon cinnamon
- 1/8 teaspoon freshly ground nutmeg
- 8 ice cubes
- Stevia to taste

Procedure:

1. Place the tea, coconut milk, nut butter, chia, protein powder, cinnamon, nutmeg, and ice cubes in a blender.
2. Process until smooth and sweeten with stevia to taste. If too thick, add ¼–½ cup water.
3. Divide into two glasses. Serve immediately.

Cinnamon Chai Smoothie

If you're a fan of coffee shop drinks with flavorful spices, you'll adore this healthier smoothie that's higher in protein and lower in sugar. Don't toss cold coffee or tea, use it to make this smoothie.

Serves 2

Ingredients:

- 1½ cups coconut milk or coconut kefir (dairy-free)
- 1½ cups iced coffee or black tea
- ¼ cup macadamia nuts or almonds
- 1 scoop plain or vanilla protein powder (choose pea, hemp, hydrolyzed beef, or hydrolyzed collagen)
- ½ teaspoon vanilla extract
- ¼ teaspoon ground cinnamon
- 8 ice cubes
- Stevia to taste

Procedure:

1. Place the coconut milk or coconut kefir, coffee, or tea, nuts, protein powder, vanilla, cinnamon, and ice cubes in a blender.
2. Process until smooth and sweeten with stevia to taste. If too thick, add ¼–½ cup water.
3. Divide into two glasses. Serve immediately.

Double Dark Chocolate Smoothie

Fiber- and nutrient-rich avocado gives this shake its thick, creamy texture. Using unsweetened organic cocoa powder ensures you get 100 percent of chocolate's flavor *and* nutrition like iron, fiber, and loads of antioxidants.

Serves 2

Ingredients:

- 1½ cups coconut milk or coconut kefir (dairy-free)
- 1 cup iced coffee or black tea
- 1 ripe avocado
- 2 tablespoons unsweetened cacao powder
- 2 tablespoons macadamia nuts or almonds
- 1 scoop plain, vanilla, or chocolate protein powder (choose pea, hemp, hydrolyzed beef, or hydrolyzed collagen)
- ½ teaspoon vanilla extract
- 1 tablespoon honey or stevia to taste
- 8 ice cubes

Procedure:

1. Place the coconut milk, iced coffee, or black tea, avocado, cacao, nuts, protein powder, honey or stevia to taste, vanilla, and ice cubes in a blender.
2. Process until smooth—if too thick, add ¼–½ cup water.

3.   Divide into two glasses. Serve immediately.

Spicy Pumpkin Pie Smoothie

Celebrate the season (any season) with this pie-inspired smoothie that's high in superfood pumpkin, rich in skin nutritive compounds like beta-carotene and tummy-filling fiber. Apple, an unsung superfood, is high in cancer fighting compounds and pectin that can help you to feel full with fewer calories.

Serves 2

Ingredients:

- 1 cup coconut milk or coconut kefir (dairy-free)
- 1 apple, quartered, cored
- ¾ cup canned pumpkin
- ¼ cup chia or hemp seeds, or 1 scoop protein powder
- 1 scoop plain or vanilla protein powder (choose pea, hemp, hydrolyzed beef, or hydrolyzed collagen)
- ½ teaspoon vanilla extract
- ½ teaspoon ground cinnamon
- 8 ice cubes
- Stevia to taste

Procedure:

1. Place the coconut milk or coconut kefir, apple, pumpkin, chia or hemp seeds, vanilla, cinnamon, 2/3 cup cold water and ice cubes, in a blender.
2. Process until smooth and sweeten with stevia to taste. If too thick, add ¼–½cup water.
3. Divide into two glasses. Serve immediately.

Chillin' Cucumber Smoothie

Cool down after a hot workout with this low-cal smoothie that can also double as a calorie friendly snack. Cucumber is high in water content, which helps to hydrate. Coconut milk contains anti-inflammatory fats that soothe, satiate, and satisfy.

Serves 2

Ingredients:

- 1 cup kale
- ½ large cucumber, peeled
- 1 ripe pear or apple, quartered, cored
- ½ cup coconut milk
- ½ cup cold green tea
- 1/3 cup hemp, pistachios, or pumpkin seeds
- 1 scoop plain or vanilla protein powder (choose pea, hemp, hydrolyzed beef, or hydrolyzed collagen)

- 8 ice cubes
- Stevia to taste

Procedure:

1. Place the kale, cucumber, pear or apple, coconut milk, green tea, seeds, and ice cubes in a blender.
2. Process until smooth and sweeten with stevia to taste.
3. Divide into two glasses. Serve immediately.

Snacks

Goji Chocolate Nut Bar

This flavorful chocolate nut bar contains healthy brain compounds from dark chocolate (for memory) and walnuts (omega-3 for detox). It also boasts a whopping 3 grams of cleansing fiber per serving that you won't find in commercial milk chocolate bars.

Serves 4

Ingredients:

- Cooking spray
- 1 cup assorted nuts, chopped
- ½ cup goji berries

- 12 ounces (2 cups) 70% dark stevia-sweetened chocolate— either Lily's® brand or Coco Polo®
- Pinch of cinnamon and cayenne
- 2 tablespoons chia seeds

Procedure:

1. Coat an 8 x 8 baking dish with wax paper. Spray the top of the wax paper, and spread around the nuts and goji berries.
2. Place the chocolate in a small saucepan over low heat and warm 2 to 3 minutes, stirring well until melted.
3. Pour over the nuts and gojis, smooth the top with a spatula.
4. Sprinkle with the chia and refrigerate at least 1 hour until firm.

Pumped Up Guacamole with Watercress and Pomegranate Arils

Watercress, rich in a long list of vitamins like A, C, and K, pumps up the nutrition in your standard guacamole. Dip in with veggies, instead of corn chips, to keep calories in check and your elimination diet on track.

Serves 4

Ingredients:

- 2 Hass avocados
- 1 cup watercress or spinach, chopped

- ¼ cup cilantro, chopped
- 1 jalapeno, seeded, minced
- 2 tablespoons minced onions
- 1 lime, juiced
- ¼ teaspoon salt
- 1 cup pomegranate arils
- 1 red pepper, thinly sliced, seeded

Procedure:

1. Place the avocado, watercress, cilantro, jalapeno, onions, lime juice, and salt in a bowl.
2. Mash the avocado mixture with the back of a wooden spoon.
3. Top with the pomegranate arils and serve immediately with the peppers.

Soups

Herby Chilled Beet Soup with Avocado

Sweet beets, a feast for the eyes, are also body-beautiful and high in folate—a heart and cancer protective compound. If you prefer the taste of cooked beets, shop for pre-steamed beets in your local grocer or roast them yourself if you desire a richer flavor.

Serves 4

Ingredients:

- 1½ pound raw beets, peeled, grated
- 1 quart homemade chicken broth
- ¼ cup chopped onion
- 2 garlic cloves, minced
- ¼ teaspoon sea salt
- ¼ teaspoon freshly ground black pepper
- ½ pound cooked shrimp or chicken
- 2 avocados, diced
- ½ cup thinly sliced radish (optional)
- ¼ cup chopped herbs

Procedure:

1. Place the beets, broth, onion, garlic, salt, and black pepper in a blender and process until smooth.
2. Divide into four bowls and top each with a 4 to 5 shrimp or sliced chicken, ½ avocado, radish, and herbs.

Watercress Almond Soup

Watercress, a spicy green that is part of the cruciferous family, gives this soup a horseradish like kick. If you are not a fan of spicy, substitute baby spinach or kale for the watercress. They are just as nutritious.

Serves 4

Ingredients:

- 4 ounces watercress
- 2 large cucumbers
- 2 avocados
- 3 cups chicken broth
- 1 cup unsweetened coconut or almond milk
- 2 tablespoons almonds
- ½ teaspoon garlic salt
- ¼ teaspoon freshly ground black pepper
- 2 cups cherry tomatoes, diced
- 2 tablespoons chopped tarragon, lemon balm, or basil
- 1 teaspoon red wine vinegar
- ¼ teaspoon salt
- 1 pound cooked shrimp or shredded chicken

Procedure:

1. Place the watercress, cucumber, avocados, chicken broth, coconut or almond milk, almonds, garlic salt, and black pepper in a blender.
2. Blend until smooth.
3. Mix the cherry tomatoes, herbs, vinegar, and salt.
4. Divide into bowls and top with the tomato mixture and shrimp or chicken. Serve immediately.

Broths

Bone Broth

Savory slow-cooked bone broth has a superior taste and a silky texture that makes the effort well worth it. Some studies show that eating bone broth may boost immunity and functional doctors prize it for its collagen content, which can soothe leaky gut and improve gut health.

Serves 8

Ingredients:

- 1 tablespoon safflower or olive oil
- 3 pounds beef marrow and knuckle bones
- 2 pounds beef shanks or oxtails or meaty bones such as short ribs
- 3 celery stalks, halved
- 3 carrots, halved
- 3 onions, quartered
- ½ cup fresh parsley stems and leaves
- Pinch of salt
- 2 tablespoons tomato paste
- ½ cup vinegar

Procedure:

1. Warm the oil in a large stockpot over medium-high heat.

2. Add the bones in batches and brown 4 to 5 minutes, turning often until they brown. Remove from pot once browned. While you brown the last batch, add the tomato paste to stockpot, reducing the heat to low. Return all the bones to the stockpot and add the vinegar and 3 quarts of water.

3. Add the celery, carrots, onions, parsley, tomato paste, and salt.

4. Add the vinegar and 3 quarts of water.

5. Bring to a boil over high heat.

6. Simmer, covered, 12 to 24 hours.

7. Alternatively, transfer it to a slow cooker and set to high for 14 hours.

8. Let the broth cool and strain it, making sure all marrow is knocked out of the bones and into the broth.

9. Serve immediately or cool completely before storing in an airtight container, refrigerated, up to a week. Or freeze for up to 6 months.

Easy Chicken Bone Broth Recipe

Ingredients:

- Whole, free-range chicken
- Apple cider vinegar
- 1 onion
- 6 peppercorns
- 3 bay leaves
- 6 cloves of garlic

- 4 carrots
- 1 bunch of celery
- 3 potatoes

Procedure:

1. Place a whole free-range chicken in your crockpot.
2. Chop all vegetables and add to pot.
3. Add spices to pot.
4. Fill the pot with cold, filtered water.
5. Add 2 tablespoons of apple cider vinegar.
6. Cook on low for 24 hours.
7. After 24 hours, remove chicken, chicken pieces, and vegetable with a slotted spoon—reserve for other dishes if desired.
8. Strain stock and reserve liquid in covered containers in your refrigerator or freezer.

Use this stock as the base of your cooking for the week—in soups, sauces, or in place of water/liquid in any other recipes.

Salads

Steak Salad with Mojo Dressing

Scrap the high calorie steak frites and dig into this steak salad that tops the charts with nutrition. Mixing proteins and superfood veggies like watercress, spinach, red bell pepper, and artichoke packs in high levels of nutrients like vitamin C, niacin, and zinc.

Serves 4

Ingredients:

- ¼ cup red or green mojo (see recipe below)
- 2 tablespoons extra virgin olive oil or coconut oil
- 1 pound watercress or spinach
- 4 large tomatoes, sliced
- 4 carrots, peeled and chopped
- ½ pound thinly sliced flank steak
- 9 ounces frozen artichokes, defrosted

Procedure:

1. Place the mojo in a small bowl along with the olive oil. Whisk well to combine and set aside.
2. Arrange the watercress or spinach, tomato, and carrot onto a platter.
3. Arrange the flank steak and artichokes on top and drizzle with mojo dressing. Serve immediately.

Red Mojo

The word mojo comes from the Spanish word for sauce. If

you've never tasted mojo you will adore this tangy sauce that gets its deep flavor from dried chilies and garlic with a lift from citrus.

Makes 1 cup

Ingredients:

- 4 dried chilies such as, ancho or arbol, stems removed, seeded
- 4 garlic cloves
- 1 teaspoon paprika
- ¼ teaspoon sea salt
- 1 cup roasted red peppers
- 2 tablespoons red wine vinegar
- ½ cup olive oil

Procedure:

1. Place the chilies in ½ cup warm water and rest for 30 minutes to hydrate them.
2. Place the garlic cloves, paprika, and salt in a food processor and process until the garlic is finely chopped.
3. Add the chilies along with their soaking water, the roasted red peppers, and vinegar. Process until the chilies are finely chopped.
4. With the motor running, add the olive oil until a thick sauce forms. Use immediately as a condiment or with any of the

recipes that call for green mojo, or store in an airtight container, refrigerated for up to 1 week.

Green Mojo

Most green mojos use cilantro as its base, a flavorful floral herb that you can find next to the parsley in the produce isle. This functional twist adds superfood spinach to boost nutrition without compromising taste.

Makes 1 cup

Ingredients:

- 3 cloves garlic, peeled
- ½ teaspoon sea salt
- 2 cups packed spinach leaves
- 1 bunch cilantro, stems trimmed
- ½ cup extra virgin olive oil

Procedure:

1. Place the garlic and salt in a food processor and chop.
2. Add the spinach and cilantro, pulsing until the greens are finely chopped.
3. With the motor running, add the olive oil in a stream until a thick sauce forms.

4. Use immediately as a condiment or with any of the recipes that call for green mojo, or store in an airtight container, refrigerated for up to 1 week.

Green Goddess Cobb

This is not your standard Cobb salad; it's powered by serious greens. Use them in the dressing to add taste and nutrition, and serve your fixings on top of superfood kale or spinach for health.

Serves 4

Ingredients:

- ½ pound nitrate-free, preferably organic bacon
- 10 ounces chopped or baby kale, any variety
- 2 large tomatoes (about 1 pound)
- 1 avocado, diced
- 4 scallions, chopped

For the dressing:

- 1 cup packed kale or spinach leaves
- 1 lemon, zested and juiced
- 2 tablespoons tahini paste
- 2 tablespoons extra virgin olive oil

- ¼ teaspoon sea salt
- 1/8 teaspoon freshly ground black pepper

Procedure:

1. Prepare the bacon per the package instructions.
2. Once cooled, chop the bacon.
3. Arrange the kale on a large platter. Top with the bacon, tomato, avocado, and scallions.
4. Prepare the dressing.
5. Place the kale or spinach, lemon zest and juice, tahini, olive oil, salt, and black pepper in a blender. Process until smooth.
6. Drizzle over salad and serve immediately.

Entrees

Ground Beef Picadillo with Lettuce Cups

Picadillo, a traditional Latin beef dish with a sweet-and-sour flare, is a fragrant chopped meat flavored with tomatoes, raisins, and olives. Use grass-fed beef for less fat and more nutrition, plus a big boost of iron. To save on grass-fed meat, shop in bulk, and store it in your freezer.

Serves 8

Ingredients:

- 2 tablespoons olive oil
- 2 pounds grass-fed ground beef
- 1 large white onion, chopped
- 8 garlic cloves, minced
- 3 bay leaves
- ¼ cup tomato paste
- 1 teaspoon mild chili powder
- ¼ teaspoon cayenne pepper
- 1 14-ounce can diced tomatoes in juice
- ¾ cup sliced, drained pimiento-stuffed green olives (from 5-ounce jar)
- ½ cup raisins
- 1 tablespoon red wine vinegar
- 1 head butter lettuce, broken into leaves (at least 12 leaves)

Procedure:

1. Warm a large stockpot over medium-high heat. Add the beef and cook 2 to 3 minutes, without breaking it up, until it browns.
2. Flip and cook 2 minutes more to brown.
3. Next, scatter the onion, garlic, and bay leaves over the browned meat, cooking until the onion is soft, about 5 minutes, breaking up the beef as the onions cook.
4. Add the tomato paste, chili, and cayenne powder, cooking one minute more until the spices become fragrant.

5. Add the diced tomatoes and their juice, olives, raisins, and vinegar.
6. Simmer until picadillo thickens, stirring occasionally, about 8 minutes.
7. Discard bay leaves.
8. Serve half the picadillo warm in lettuce cups and reserve the remainder for leftovers.

Grilled Salmon with Pineapple Cilantro Salsa

Juicy sweet pineapple is the perfect foil for fatty rich salmon. Asparagus, the ideal veggie partner with salmon adds a colorful green base along with prebiotic fiber for optimal gut health.

Serves 4

Ingredients:

- 1 cup cubed pineapple, finely chopped
- ½ green bell pepper or poblano chili, diced
- ¼ red onion, diced (about 1/4 cup)
- 2 tablespoons fresh cilantro leaves, chopped
- 1 lime, zested and juiced
- ½ teaspoon salt, divided
- 1/8teaspoon ground cayenne or paprika
- 1 pound wild salmon filets, skin removed

- 1 tablespoon Sriracha
- 1 pound asparagus, trimmed

Procedure:

1. Prepare the salsa. Place the pineapple, pepper, onion, cilantro, lime zest and juice, half the salt, and cayenne or paprika in a small bowl, toss well.
2. Preheat the grill over high heat. Sprinkle the salmon with the remaining salt and spread the Sriracha over top.
3. Place the salmon and asparagus on the grill and cook 4 to 5 minutes for the asparagus, turning the salmon once. Continue to cook the salmon 3 to 4 minutes more until it is still pink but no longer translucent.
4. Serve immediately with the asparagus and the salsa.

Buffalo Burger in a Napa Wrap

Serves 4

Ingredients:

- 1 pound ground buffalo or bison meat
- ¼ teaspoon sea salt
- 1 tablespoons coconut or avocado oil
- 4 large Napa cabbage leaves
- 1 large tomato, thinly sliced

- 8 pickles (optional)
- 4 tablespoons organic, sugar-free ketchup, mojo, or eggless, soy-free mayo (I love Sir Kensington's Fabanaise egg-free, soy-free vegan mayo for the elimination diet. It comes in plain or chipotle.)
- 1 head broccoli, cut into 4 large florets

Procedure:

1. Prepare the burgers. Mix the meat with the salt and form into 4 patties.
2. Heat a large skillet over high heat, add the oil and the burgers and cook 10 to 12 minutes, turning occasionally until the burgers are medium-rare.
3. Wrap each burger in a cabbage leaf and top with the pickles, ketchup, or soy-free, egg-free mayo.
4. While the burgers are cooking, fill a large stockpot with 1 inch of water and bring to a boil over high.
5. Add the broccoli and steam 4 to 5 minutes until fork tender.
6. Once cooked and plated, drizzle with olive oil and salt.
7. Serve immediately with burgers.

EVERYTHING YOU NEED TO KNOW TO MAKE GREEN DRINKS AND SMOOTHIES ON YOUR OWN

Once you get the hang of it, green drinks and smoothies are easy to make, and the combinations are endless. Below is a simple framework that you can follow.

Step 1: Choose your base

Add 2 cups of one of the following bases to your blender:

- Water
- Coconut water
- Coconut milk
- Almond milk
- Cashew milk
- Hemp milk
- Bulgarian or sheep's milk yogurt and kefir—allowed post-elimination diet for those without dairy sensitivities

Step 2: Choose your greens

Choose 2 cups (tightly packed) of the following greens and add to your blender:

- Spinach
- Kale
- Swiss chard
- Collard greens
- Dandelion greens
- Turnip greens

- Beet greens
- Sweet potato greens
- Romaine lettuce
- Spring mix

Step 3: Choose your fruit

Choose ½ cup–1 cup of the following fruit to add to your blender:

- Banana
- Cherries
- Raspberries
- Blueberries
- Blackberries
- Strawberries
- Mango
- Pineapple
- Papaya
- Avocado
- Peaches
- Pears
- Apples

Step 4: Add your protein

Choose 1 scoop of the following protein powders:

- Pea protein isolate
- Hemp protein powder
- Hydrolyzed beef protein powder
- Hydrolyzed collagen powder

Step 5: Supercharge it

Choose 1 tablespoon of the following superfoods to add to your blender:

- Coconut oil
- Cacao
- Chia seeds
- Hemp seeds
- Cinnamon
- Vanilla
- Maca
- Spirulina
- Chlorella

Blend and enjoy!

Will yield roughly 32 ounces, which may equate to 1–2 servings.

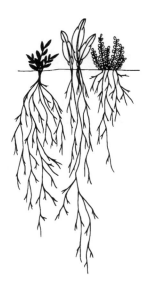

CHAPTER 4

Step 3: ROOT— Gratitude, Connection, and Restoration

———

In Step 2, we took a huge leap in this process by learning how to use nutrition and primary foods to create the ideal conditions for your seeds of desire to flourish. In Step 3, we will address one of the most neglected aspects of cultivating sustainable health: becoming rooted, connected, and anchored in your life.

What does this mean? Just as a plant must be firmly rooted before it can grow to its full potential, you must also put down roots so you can grow strong and cultivate focus to accomplish your health and life goals and achieve full Bloom.

LET'S START BY TALKING ABOUT YOUR DAY

Let me take a guess at what your average day is like. You wake up (or are woken up) feeling tired, maybe you press the snooze button a few times before rushing out of bed to grab a BIG cup of coffee to energize you for the long day ahead.

For those with children, this dreaded time of day is often referred to as the "morning crush," characterized by trying to get everyone up, dressed, fed, and out the door in an insanely short amount of time. As a mother of two young children, I feel frazzled just thinking about it.

Once you're done with that fiasco, it's time to fight traffic to get to work on time, where you are greeted with piles of emails, messages, and deadlines. You may have to deal with unhappy clients, put out fires around the office, and play counselor to staff and co-workers. Perhaps you slip away to take a lunch break, but many people do not.

After eight or more long hours, you leave work, pick up your kids (if you have them), rush them to and from after school activities, and (finally) head home to make dinner. Maybe you try and squeeze in a workout or walk the dog, but it's already evening, the kids need help with their homework, and you would *love* to spend a few meaningful moments with your partner—or yourself—before the "bedtime crush." After that, you help with clean up and try to get everyone in bed by a sane hour.

By now, it's probably near nine o'clock, at which time you have more emails, text messages, bills, school stuff, and other grown-up things to attend to. Maybe you have time to read or relax before bed, but by now you're pretty spent and you just want to go to sleep. It has been another stressful, no-time-for-anything day, and you're going to have to do it again tomorrow, so you lie awake thinking about it.

If this sounds insane, that's because it is! In a typical day like this, there is no time to recharge your batteries or stop to reflect. This lifestyle, compounded daily, has a deleterious effect on our bodies and our souls. Instinctually, you know this is not healthy and wish it were different. I see it take shape in my patients in the form of anxiety, fatigue, insomnia, digestive disorders, stress, and burnout.

Days like these can feel even more overwhelming if you have additional responsibilities such as children, caring for a parent or loved one, or uneven distribution of tasks in a relationship or household.

How much time does this leave for you to work on your health, desires, and recharge your batteries? Zero, zilch, nada. However, things weren't always this way for women. As we learned in Chapter 3, in hunter-gatherer societies, food gathering and preparation took up a small part of the day, leaving ample time for taking care of children, socializing, and working on other chores in a community setting.

This is not to say we should aspire to spend our lives solely meal planning, housekeeping, and entertaining; but it does illustrate that missing aspect of tribe, support, and belonging among women. Even our mothers' generation—with their bridge clubs, church groups, and more balanced work schedules—had better built-in support systems than we do. We have made many cultural and technological advances, of course, but some wonderful parts of our culture is gone, and it stings.

FIGHT, FLIGHT, AND HEALING

When I talk to patients about their lifestyles, nearly all of them convey the feeling of "barely surviving" at life, physically and emotionally. They are exhausted, inflamed, and fed up with the imbalance of responsibilities in their lives. Who can blame them? Today's always-on, twenty-four-seven, data-driven world demands a heck of a lot from us, and it takes its toll.

One of the ways modern stress affects our health is by trapping us in what is known as a *sympathetic autonomic nervous system response*, also known as "fight or flight."

When our body responds this way, we secrete neurotransmitters that cause our adrenal glands to produce the stress hormones: epinephrine and cortisol. These stress hormones send the message to our body: "You are in danger!" When this message is received, the body responds by increasing blood pressure and heart rate, wound healing halts, and our sex drive, digestion, and immune system shutdown to divert energy to fighting or flighting, while our adrenaline soars.[1] This is a natural and beneficial evolutionary process for survival, but we are not meant to dwell in fight-or-flight mode long term, and the side effects of excess epinephrine, cortisol, and elevated adrenaline levels are detrimental to our health.

Conversely, when we are relaxed and balanced, we are living in what is known as *parasympathetic mode*, also known as the "direct-or-digest" response. This causes our blood pressure to decrease and our pulse to slow down. It also supports digestion through the vagus nerve, discussed in the previous chapter, which supports the muscles of sexual arousal, keeps our immune system humming along, and maintains full body balance.[2] Humans are meant to live this way; this is normal, but we live in a very skewed world where everything is a crisis.

Ultimately, this state of being leaves us vulnerable to acute and chronic diseases, mental and emotional imbalance, and does not allow us to take in nourishment for our seeds to grow and maintain strong roots. It un-grounds us, body and soul, and is not sustainable for long-term health.

In Step 3, we will focus on practical implementation of specific guiding principles that will interrupt and replace this chronic fight-or-flight cycle with a healthier, grounded response to stress. *Practical* is the key word here, because let's be real, *we have the world we have* and it's going to be busy, stressful, and at times, darn right difficult. Therefore, if we have any hope of creating strong, grounded roots, we must create a reservoir of restoration—think of it as your emergency stash of health for when life's storms hit. If your typical day is anything like the previously described vignette, you can bet your current reservoir is bone dry.

BUCKET THEORY

I often tell my patients to think about building their reservoirs using this "Bucket Theory":

Imagine you have two buckets. One is your stress bucket and the other is your happy bucket. To encourage good health, you always want to have more in your happy bucket than your stress bucket. How do you rebalance the distribution in your buckets? By taking time to take care of YOU. You have already given yourself permission to do so in Chapter 1, and now I am going to hold you to it. This chapter will give you exercises, tools, and tips on how to build and maintain a self-care regime that will fill your happy bucket and give you a bottomless reservoir of restoration.

BUILD YOUR SANCTUARY

A sanctuary, or sacred space, is a quiet and inspiring physical place for practicing daily rituals, setting intentions, reflecting, and centering. Since all these restorative practices are crucial to filling your reservoir of health, we are going to go through the steps of creating your own sanctuary now.

Start by choosing a peaceful place where you can be alone to replenish yourself, clear your mind, reflect, reconnect, and anchor yourself in parasympathetic or "restorative" mode. Using an indoor space could mean dedicating an entire room of your home or a little corner of a room; it could mean carving out a spot on your bookshelf or setting up a little table. If you feel more grounded outdoors, you can set aside a space in your garden, screened porch, or your yard.

Next, let's talk décor. How you design your sanctuary matters—it should be a place that is comfortable and pleasing enough to spend five minutes or five hours—so less is more here. Aim for a décor that's simple, peaceful, beautiful, calming, and centering such as:

- Flowers
- Crystals
- Stones
- Feathers
- Pictures of your family and places you love
- Religious or spiritual art
- An essential oil diffuser
- A space for journaling with your journal, pen, etc., at hand
- A chair, pillow, or yoga mat for meditation
- A comfortable throw
- Art supplies

After selecting a spot, preparing, and decorating your sacred space, plan on spending some time with it every day. Your sanctuary is a material manifestation of that permission to care for yourself, your anchor point to your intentions and goals, so it is important you make it part of your daily routine. For those of us with busy schedules, it's best to carve out a set time in the morning, before the day begins, or schedule a time at night as things are winding down.

One final note on building your sanctuary: In the interest of unplugging and embracing solitude, your sacred space should remain an electronic-free zone. Exceptions would be using a device to play relaxation music, a motivational message, or guided meditation; in which case, I suggest putting the device on "Do Not Disturb" or "Airplane Mode" to avoid any distractions.

CONSTRUCTING YOUR SANCTUARY: THREE EASY STEPS

1. Choose a place in your home or outdoors where you can get a little bit of quiet space.

2. Decorate (not clutter) the space sparingly with things that remind you of how you want to feel and grow in your life.

3. Spend time there every single day.

Though it may seem like another new trend in the personal development world, adopting an "attitude of gratitude" has become popular for a darn good reason: It works. More specifically, it has been proven to impact your life and health in profoundly positive ways.

Emotionally, cultivating gratitude connects us with something larger than ourselves, thereby allowing us to live a more joyful life and relate to people in a more meaningful and positive way. From a health and healing perspective, gratitude constitutes a counterbalance against the physical and cognitive limitations of disease. In other words, gratitude allows us to be more resilient.

Gratitude also provides the following health benefits:

- Plays a major role in improving quality of life;[3]
- Correlated with positive emotional functioning, lower dysfunction, and more positive social relationships;[4]
- Reduces inflammatory biomarkers;[5]
- Decreases stress, thereby helping you switch to parasympathetic mode (aka restoration mode);[6]
- Improves heart rate variability;[4] and
- Lowers fatigue and improves sleep quality.[7]

In other words, it is physiological and biochemical magic.

GRATITUDE JOURNALING

One of the easiest ways to strengthen your roots and get grounded is to keep a gratitude journal.

This practice of focusing on small things for which you are grateful—the sky, the birds, a comfortable bed, good food, your new nail polish—shifts perspective and attitude very quickly.

Let's try it out right now. Set a timer for two minutes and write down ten things you are grateful for. Remember, they need not be large or grandiose, just anything that makes your heart rejoice.

1.

2.

3.

4.

5.

6.

7.

8.

9.

10.

There—don't you feel better already? Now, if you can make a point to write in your gratitude journal every single day, it *will* change your life. Keep your journal in your sanctuary, and write in it there every day.

As of this writing in 2017, there have been numerous studies showing that connection to others is good for our health and longevity. A 2010 meta-analysis of 148 studies on the longevity effects of social relationships performed by professors at Brigham Young University in Utah, concluded those with strong social relationships have a whopping 50 percent lower chance of mortality than those without.[8] Conversely, a 2015 study published in the *British Medical Journal* showed that feelings of loneliness and social isolation increased a person's risk of heart disease, America's number one killer, by 29 percent.[9]

Further, in his book, *Healthy at 100,*[10] John Robbins talks a great deal about the emphasis on connection and community in the different cultures he studied with great longevity. Friendship literally keeps us alive.

I have seen the importance of friendship play out in my own life and in the lives of my loved ones. My grandmother, for example, lived to be 103 years old, and for ninety of those years, she and her best friend were there for each other through thick and thin. They met when they were teenagers, and their friendship supported my grandmother, as she made it through school and got her PhD in the 1940s. They both left Cuba after the Revolution and came to the United States in their late fifties. Their friendship saw them both through difficult times, and, even after their deaths, has affected subsequent generations.

Friendship is important for everyone, yet I see an epidemic of social isolation in my female patients, especially those with children. The study titled "UCLA Study On Friendship Among Women" found, whenever women get busy with life, family, etc., their friendships with other women are the first thing to be let go. The problem with that, per the study, is women provide a real source of strength for one another, in the way they talk with and relate to one another. Take away that strength, and we tend to become weaker without it.[11]

This goes back to that making-time-for-self thing we keep talking about. When we're young and unattached, it's easy to spend a lot of time with friends, but that changes as we grow up and the responsibilities pile up. For our generation of working women especially, it can be guilt-inducing to spend what little free time we have away from our children. However, if you are serious about cultivating health, then you must get serious about cultivating real friendships. Plus, it is an excellent opportunity to set a good example of friendship for your children, because they need to learn that through their parents.

Case in point, a 2006 study of 3,000 nurses with breast

cancer found women without close friends were four times more likely to die from breast cancer as women with ten or more friends.[12] If you're wondering how *anyone* has time to see ten (or more) friends on a regular basis, you will be relieved to learn the proximity of the friends wasn't associated with survival. In other words, these women's friends weren't necessarily people they could meet up with for coffee, but people with whom they had developed deep connections. The mere fact of having friends, regardless of their location, is protective.

That said, it is vitally important to choose friends that lift you up and inspire you, because the people you spend time with have a tremendous influence on your life experience.

There are many important connections we make in life, and it is important to foster them. Your deepest and most lasting relationship is, of course, to yourself, and much of this book is dedicated to nurturing the health and development of that relationship. It is also critical to build and nourish relationships with friends. Push for your friendships. Make a point to spend time with your friends on a regular basis, and the rewards will be lifelong.

Think about your happiest times in your life: falling in love, traveling, becoming a parent, celebrating a big career advancement, accomplishing a huge life's goal, etc. More likely than not, those were not solitary experiences, rather shared times with friends, family, and loved ones. It is *shared* experiences that bring the greatest joy and happiness.

SPIRITUALITY

Spirituality is the way we experience our connectedness to the moment, to self, to others, to nature, and to the significant and sacred. It is also the way we express meaning in our lives. Taking the time to connect to the divine, or something larger than ourselves, has proven a key component to creating better health outcomes.

For example, spiritual well-being has shown to have significant bearing on the quality of life among cancer patients. It was even more important than physical well-being, social and family well-being, and emotional well-being.

Spirituality, in the context of creating your root system, is fundamentally about being connected to the divine—or something larger than yourself—so you have something or someone to turn to when challenges arise. Analyses have shown spiritual or religious practice played a considerable role in mortality rate reductions—so significant a role it was deemed comparable to fruit and vegetable consumption and cholesterol therapy.[13]

When counseling patients on the importance of spirituality in healing, many of them fondly reminisce about the comforting rituals and routines they experienced growing up in religious or spiritual families. Yet, as they grew up, they found life got too busy for them to engage in their spiritual side.

Since spiritual practices produce such a robust array of benefits, I typically recommend patients take steps to reconnect to a spiritual practice. Whether that means spending time in prayer and communion with a specific divinity, joining a meditation class, or going for a hike in the woods, seeking out spiritual connection is a vital step in becoming rooted in your health goals and life's purpose.

Now, let me be clear that I understand finding a religious path may not be right for everyone, especially those who have purposefully cast off past religious or spiritual affiliations because of specific disagreements with doctrine, abusive practices, or simply due to a lack of spiritual fulfillment. If this is the case, I would encourage you, instead, to nurture your spirituality through meaningful, regular connections with your community, spending time in nature or meditation, and to take steps to serve a purpose larger than yourself, which studies have suggested may also increase longevity[14] and help you feel better in your body.

JULIA'S STORY

Julia was raised in a very Catholic household. She prayed regularly and attended church with her family every week. When she met her husband, he was also very spiritual, and they were on the same page religiously for some time. As the years went by, he got busy with work and stopped going to church, and then, after a while, so did she.

Down the road, she ended up experiencing struggles with her marriage, her career, and her body. During a consultation, Julia and I had an in-depth conversation about spirituality, and she realized she truly missed having a spiritual practice in her life. Up until then, she had been unaware of how much its absence affected her, but once she realized it, everything changed. She found a church that resonated with her beliefs and attended regularly. Within a few weeks, her anxiety decreased, her marriage was improving, she made new friendships, her career struggles lessened, and she saw great improvements in her health.

Keep in mind not everyone will practice spirituality in the same way. For some, it means attending church. For others, it is being out in nature, connecting through art, crystals, meditation, prayers, music, or other spiritual rituals. Almost any form of divine-focused expression—from singing and dancing to everyday conversations—can be treated as a spiritual practice. Think about what you like to do, and how it manifests the divine for you.

NINE SIMPLE WAYS TO FILL YOUR
SPIRITUAL RESERVOIR

- Sing or chant mantras—research has shown that when you sing simple song structures, or when you hum or chant mantras, prayers, or hymns, you increase your heart rate variability, which triggers your parasympathetic nervous system response.[15]

- Do some artwork.

- Meditate—meditation and prayer have both been shown to have a positive impact on how our genes are expressed (known as epigenetics).[16]

- Pray.

- Play a musical instrument.

- Spend time appreciating nature.

- Attend religious or spiritual services.

- Help others.

- Read about spirituality, the sacred, or other self-improvement literature.

Finally, in pursuing a relationship with the sacred, it is important not only to focus your intentions on the divine but also to *practice*. Creating a sanctuary space, as we discussed, is a good place to start. From there, be sure and take the time to practice gratitude journaling, quiet meditation, prayers, or saying a mantra every single day. This constant practice will re-pattern your brain to adopt a more optimistic, calm, and rooted state of mind, which will positively affect your health and well-being.

TOP THREE RESTORATIVE CONNECTIONS

1. Connection to yourself.

2. Connection to others.

3. Connection to the divine or something larger than yourself.

RESTORING YOURSELF

The most important restorative activity for health is one we do (hopefully) every day: *sleep*.

It seems like such a simple need to meet, yet we try to get by with way less sleep than our bodies require. We have become so busy staying connected and productive that we don't honor or value restoration anymore. Some people even think of the need to rest and sleep as a weakness, when it is *imperative* to our health—and, ironically, our ability to be productive in the first place.

Undoubtedly, there are circumstances when we must sacrifice sleep. I remember as a new mother fighting the urge to yell at every "expert" who preached about the health detriments of getting less than nine hours sleep a night (don't these people have kids?). However, even if you have a newborn or young children, you shouldn't sacrifice your sleep when you can help it.

Sleep is when your body repairs itself, assimilates nutrients, and when you engage in what has been called "synaptic pruning," the process in which your brain breaks down old information to make space for new information to integrate.[17]. When we don't allow ourselves enough sleep, it can cause our brains to feel overwhelmed by information or unable to take in new information. New mothers, for example, may experience the effects of this in the form of "mommy brain."

How much sleep do you need, and how do you prioritize it against your other needs? I tell patients to aim for seven and a half to nine hours of sleep a night, and that sleep should always be your top priority. Sleep must come first, before super-early workouts, before lengthy meditation sessions, before nearly everything else; sleep should always come first.

THE KEYS TO SLEEPING BETTER

It is all well and good to tell people to get more sleep. Many of my patients, however, struggle not only to find time to sleep but to get good quality sleep. Here are my top tips for sleeping better at night:

- Do not drink caffeine after 2:00 p.m.
- Avoid screens and bright lights for an hour or two before bed. If you must work on a device, use blue block glasses (see resource section at the end of the chapter).

- Avoid alcohol before bed. Though it can have a temporarily sedative effect, the sugar can keep you up.
- Get your exercise in early, preferably before evening, or it can amp you up.
- Set boundaries throughout your day. For example, two hours before bed make a point to start winding down and being incommunicado.
- If you tend to get revved up in the evenings, channel that energy into gardening or taking a walk with your family after dinner.
- Take advice from those baby books and give yourself a bedtime ritual. Once you've powered down for the day, make a cup of chamomile, lemon balm, or valerian tea, or take an Epsom salt bath. Then spend a few minutes in your sanctum praying, meditating, and putting the day to rest.
- Try journaling before bed. This helps get the day's thoughts, worries, and excitement out of your head and prepares the space for tomorrow.
- Make your bedroom completely dark. This stimulates natural production of melatonin, your body's master sleep hormone.
- Aim for your bedroom temperature to be somewhere around 65 degrees Fahrenheit.
- If you find yourself waking up at night, try eating a small, protein-rich snack before bed. This will prevent blood sugar crashes that may cause night waking.

Natural Sleep Remedies

- Magnesium—500 mg of magnesium daily has been shown to improve common symptoms of insomnia.[18]
- Passionflower tea—has been traditionally used as a sleep aid and been shown to improve sleep quality in health adults.[19]
- Chamomile tea—is one of the most consumed herbal teas in the world for good reason, historical use and modern science tells us it helps relax the nervous system and promote sound sleep.[20]
- Valerian tincture or tea—widely used as a natural sleep aid in Europe, Valerian is a safe and natural relaxant herb that can help you get to sleep easier.[21]

EARTHING—THE ULTIMATE ROOTING PRACTICE

Earthing, also known as "grounding," is the practice of connecting with the earth's surface with your bare feet or bare skin. This simple process of walking around barefoot, gardening, walking on the beach, etc., grounds and balances your body's electrical systems in a profound way.[22]

If this sounds a little out there, remember our bodies are as much (if not more) electrical in nature as they are biological. Our brains, nervous systems, and heartbeats all function through electrical impulses—that is what's being measured when you have an EKG, for example.

Human beings, and the electronics we love, naturally emit a positive electrical charge, while the earth below us emits a natural negative charge; put the two together and you get a harmoniously balanced circuit. Direct contact with the earth also exposes us to naturally occurring antioxidant electrons shown to produce a myriad of health benefits.[23] Human beings were made to have regular contact with the earth, through our footsteps, sleeping on the ground, foraging, harvesting, swimming, etc., but we have lost regular contact due to modern life.

Some of the proven health benefits of earthing include:

- Reduced cardiovascular risk;[24]
- Decreased blood glucose in patients with diabetes;[25]
- Improved thyroid function, including a decrease in thyroid hormone and increase in TSH;[26]
- Reduction in muscle damage after a strenuous workout;[27]
- Decreased risk factors for osteoporosis;[24]
- Improvements in sleep;[28] and,
- Improved heart rate variability and stress reduction.[29]

Beyond physical contact with the earth, studies have shown that looking at nature can bring down your stress levels,[30] and neighborhoods with ample trees and greenspace have improved mental health outcomes and lower rates of violent crime.[31]

The easiest way to get more earthing and nature into your life is to walk around your yard barefoot every day (walking barefoot on concrete counts too). Or, if you are able, take your work outside, and engage in as many outdoor activities as possible. Gardening is another fantastic way to simultaneously soothe yourself, spend time earthing, and beautify your environment. Habitual gardeners have also been shown to have better wellness outcomes, such as less stress, better focus, pain control,[32] as well as living longer lives.[33] Camping is a great way to spend time looking at and in touch with nature, and if you can go camping for two weeks and leave your digital devices at home, you may find your insomnia disappears. The Japanese call this "forest bathing," where you spend time in nature and allow it to wash away your stress.[34]

You can also purchase earthing mats and sheets that ground you to the earth via a copper wire. These can be hugely beneficial for those with sleeping problems or those unable to spend enough time outdoors. See the resources section at the end of this chapter for more information.

HEALING SMARTER

It can be genuinely overwhelming to consider all the avenues available for self-care and healing. However, remember, *our goal is to work smarter on your health, not harder*. You can heal smarter by doing LESS, when you switch your state of mind.

Part of the reason I love gardening is it allows me to work incredibly efficiently on my health. Since it's a physical activity, it makes me move my body, while I practice earthing and spending time in solitude or with loved ones. It also allows me space to reflect and connect to myself and nature while appreciating something divinely beautiful. Plus, I use my garden as a source of clean and nourishing vegetables, fruits, and herbs. So, by practicing one little self-care hobby, I wind up nurturing myself in multiple ways at one time.

What hobbies do you enjoy that can help you heal smarter and faster?

ESSENTIAL PHYSICAL BODY RESTORATION TECHNIQUES

There are many ways to help restore your body to a naturally fluid, flexible, toned, vibrant, and pain-free state. Some of these involve movement and some require stillness. Aim to incorporate a few of these activities into your life on a regular basis.

Massage—touch is very healing and can help destress and detoxify you while relieving muscle tension and soreness. Massages can also incorporate elements of aromatherapy to trigger a deep and healing relaxation response.

Bathing—here are my top bathing-for-health recommendations:

- Epsom salt float tanks are great for solitary relaxation (provided you don't suffer from claustrophobia).
- Swimming is vigorous and extremely restorative for the body. If you can swim in a natural, non-chlorinated body of water, like a lake, spring, or the ocean—even better!
- At-home Epsom salt/dead sea salt baths or relaxing in a salt-water hot tub are linked to a reduction in inflammation[35] which can help with eczema,[36] arthritis, and muscle aches.

Salt Rooms—these relaxation rooms are covered in Himalayan salt crystals. The experience is comparable to time spent at the beach breathing in the salty air. Salt rooms may also provide additional benefits for those with asthma and seasonal allergies.[37]

Spa Days—I often advise my patients to book a half day at the spa every couple of months. It's a great way to relax, have time alone, feel cared for and nurtured, get rooted, and refill your reservoir. If cost is an issue, look for spas that offer an amenities or spa-pass that gives you access to self-serve modalities like saunas, aromatherapy showers, salt rooms, soaking tubs, steam rooms, cold plunge pools, etc., for a low price.

Though these restorative practices may feel "indulgent" at first, remember they are essential to filling your reservoir so you can maintain good health.

EPSOM SALT BATH RECIPE

Add two cups of Epsom salts to a tub full of warm water.

Soak and enjoy for at least thirty minutes.

Tip: For added therapeutic benefits, try adding ten to twenty drops of any of the following pure essential oils: lavender, mandarin, clary sage, geranium, frankincense, vetiver, or bergamot.

GET MOVING!

Sitting has been called "the new smoking," because a sedentary lifestyle has proven detrimental to our health.

Our bodies are meant to *move*. Note I say "move" and not "exercise," because we are meant to be in motion most of the time, rather than moving intensely for a short period. Don't get me wrong, I encourage exercise, but I also encourage incorporating as much natural movement into your days as possible.

My grandmother, who lived to be 103, never exercised a day in her life; she just didn't drive a car, therefore, she walked everywhere. In the modern world, we sit at desks all day working on computers, playing on our phones, driving in cars, and we don't move as we are designed to.

Beyond our physical health, movement is good for our mental well-being and can be used to connect, to pray, and to express yourself.[38]

The best way to move more is to become *intentional* about it and plant those seeds of movement. A Fitbit®, Jawbone®, Apple Watch™, or other tracking device can be of great value in quantifying our movement. I was shocked when I began using a Fitbit and realized I wasn't moving nearly as much as I thought I was. Even without a device, you can still incorporate more movement in your life by parking farther away, taking the stairs, switching to a standing or treadmill desk, and getting a couple of little walks in whenever you can. Aim to take at least 12,000 steps per day.

I'm also a HUGE fan of dance as a joyful form of exercise, expression, and connection.

Every culture dances in some way for some reason. You can put music on and dance by yourself, take an aerobic-style dance class, or get your girlfriends together to go out dancing and let it work its delightful, mood-lifting magic.

However you choose to do it, make it a point to move more throughout your day.

WHAT DOES A HEALTHY FITNESS ROUTINE LOOK LIKE?

Your fitness routine should be enjoyable and need not mirror that of a star athlete or supermodel. Aim for forty-five minutes of moderate exercise at least three times per week. This could include any combination of movement you enjoy, including:

- Dance

- Megaformer™ training

- Total Twitch Twitch Training (t3 Approach)

- Spinning

- High Intensity Interval Training

- Pilates

- Yoga

- Running

- Interval training

- Walking

- Suspension training

- Barre

- Weight lifting

- Circuit training

- Swimming

- Resistance bands, etc.

BIOFEEDBACK

Biofeedback, an electronic way to monitor and control your autonomic nervous system response, has been one of the most effective tools in helping me, and many of my patients, stay rooted, focused, and calm.

The biofeedback tool I recommend to all my patients is called Inner Balance™, by HeartMath. It works via smartphone or computer to retrain your nervous system to quickly switch to a restorative/parasympathetic response when you default to fight or flight. It works by tracking your heart rate variability and cueing you to use your breath to return to that balanced state. It's portable, quick (most cycles only take three minutes), and easy to practice whenever you feel stressed.

Biofeedback can also help ease depression, anxiety, muscle tension, and fatigue[39] in as little as a month or two.

A STORY FROM MY ROOTS

I come from a Cuban and Mexican background; my people are joyful and dance a lot, well into old age. When my Abuela came to the United States from Cuba in 1967, she was already in her late fifties, and my grandfather was in his sixties. They were dedicated civil servants and always wanted to help, so they began to volunteer at the Little Havana Activity Center.

Every weekday, until she was well into her nineties, my grandmother volunteered there. That was her connection, and that was her community—it was so vibrant.

In the summers, when I was growing up, the Little Havana Activity Center would rent out a hotel in Miami Beach (this was back when it was still rundown, not the trendy Miami Beach we know today) and all the seniors would get to spend the summer at the beach.

I would go every year with my parents to visit my grandparents there. Most of my childhood memories of summer include hanging out with eighty-five-year-old Cuban immigrants on the beach. We would swim every morning, and the elders would sing while we swam. In the evenings, my mom would play old Cuban songs on the piano for them, and every night, those eighty-five-year-olds would dance their hearts out. There was so much joy and so much laughter on those vacations.

That kind of connection and community is a missing element in our modern society. The questions we face now are: How do we recreate that? How do we remember these ways to connect to one another and connect to our roots that we have forgotten?

By applying Step 3's guiding principles to becoming rooted—sanctuary, gratitude, friendships, spirituality, restoration, sleep, earthing, and movement—you are well on your way to establishing a strong root system that will sustain you as we dig deeper in Step 4: Weed. As always, remember to work smarter, not harder, by utilizing the resources available to you at nourishmedicine.com/bloomresources.

Root Action Items:

- Create your sanctuary in a room, on a shelf, in your garden, wherever you can find a quiet place to unplug and connect in solitude.
- Begin keeping a gratitude journal, and write in it every day.
- Make sleep your number one priority. Follow the suggestions described and aim to be in bed by 9:00 or 10:00 p.m. every night so you can get seven and a half to nine hours of quality sleep.
- Spend time in nature and give earthing a try—either spending time outside barefoot, gardening, or using an earthing mat (see resources below).
- Make it a point to reconnect, or make new connections, with female friends.
- Ask yourself, "How can I help others harvest and share their gifts?"
- Take an honest inventory of your spiritual health, and, if you haven't already, develop a regular practice of connecting with the divine.
- Incorporate joyful movement into your life every day.
- Schedule some time for one (or more) of the essential physical body restoration techniques discussed in this chapter, such as a spa day, Epsom salt bath, or massage.
- And remember to work smarter, not harder, at becoming rooted. Figure out clever ways of incorporating several of these practices into one practice, like gardening, exercising outdoors with friends, attending church, or joining a meditation group, etc.

ROOT Resources at nourishmedicine.com/bloomresources:

- Online recommendations for earthing products, HeartMath Biofeedback tools, Chilipads
- Links to crystals, journals, altars, and "sacred space" décor.

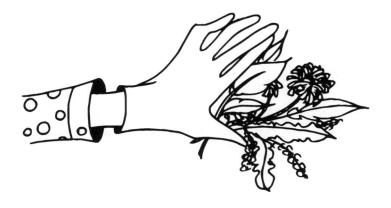

CHAPTER 5

Step 4: WEED— Toxicity

Since you are officially over half way into your Bloom journey, let's pause to reflect on the steps we have taken to reclaim your health, cultivate your desires, and reignite your spark. After preparing the fertile soil of your attitude, mind, and heart, we moved onto Step 1, where we carefully selected and sowed your seeds of desire; Step 2 taught us how to nourish them through individualized nutrition and primary foods; and in Step 3 we got grounded by strengthening your roots and balancing the stress response with self-care principles. Now that you have gained enough strength in body, mind, and spirit, it's time for Step 4: It's time to weed.

As any gardener knows, weeds are tricky, because they can pop up and take over at unexpected times and require our awareness, patience, and vigilance to control naturally. The same goes for controlling toxic influences in our lives. If we don't stay on top of identifying and weeding them regularly, they can quickly take over our health by crowding out the good stuff.

This chapter will teach you the most effective natural weed-control techniques for nipping sneaky toxins in the bud, including where to find them (they are hidden in the strangest places), how to identify them, how to get rid of them, and what to replace them with for better health.

A GOOD HARD LOOK AT THE TOXIC WORLD WE HAVE

To say we live in a toxic world would be a gross understatement.

Since World War II, per the National Toxicology Program at the United States Department of Health and Human Services, there have been over 85,000 synthetic chemicals registered with the United States Environmental Protection Agency. Every year, an estimated 2,000 new chemicals are introduced into the market for use in food, personal care products, household cleaners, pesticides, lawn care products, and nearly everything we come into daily contact with.[1] The Environmental Working Group (EWG) estimates there are about 3,000 synthetic chemicals manufactured in high production every year, and more than 1,000,000 pounds of these chemicals are produced or imported into the United States.[2]

A recent study found 167 chemical pollutants in blood and urine from test subjects, including an average of fifty-three carcinogens in each person, and the study subjects didn't live in high-pollution areas or close to industrial facilities. A 2004 study showed 287 chemicals in the umbilical cord blood of babies taken at birth, including pesticides, consumer product ingredients, and waste pollutants, as well as over 180 carcinogens.[3]

Plus, per EWG, more than 1,400 chemicals and chemical groups are known as likely carcinogens.[4]

As Americans, we are exposed daily to these cancer-causing compounds, which destroy the body and build up in the blood and urine over time.

One of the most insidious toxic weeds we encounter daily is plastic. You are probably familiar with Bisphenol A, commonly known as BPA, a powerful endocrine-disrupting chemical that mimics estrogen, resulting in negative effects on the thyroid and metabolism, and is linked to cancer, infertility, and diabetes.[5] The effects of endocrine disruptors, like BPA, fall disproportionately on young girls, as it has been suggested they are pushing them into early puberty.[6] In light of these findings, we stopped using BPA in favor of BPS, but we're seeing now that it's just as bad.[7] Unfortunately, these kinds of chemicals are pervasive—every time you go to the grocery store and are given a receipt, you are exposed to BPA in the paper. The same kind of thing happens with pesticides and flame retardants on our clothes. The stuff is *everywhere.*

Pesticides are of particular concern for parents, as they have been linked to an increased risk of cancer in children,[8] and there's mounting evidence that chronic moderate pesticide exposure is neurotoxic and increases the risk of neurological ailments such as Parkinson's Disease.[9] Because of this kind of evidence, more people are trying to commit to an organic diet, which will make a big difference, but does not take into account exposure to home toxins and indoor use of pesticides.

THREE WORST EFFECTS OF
TOXIC BODY BURDEN

- Endocrine disruption.
- Cancer-causing properties.
- Potential for transgenerational damage.

The most common toxins we are exposed to are:

- Pesticides
- Plasticizers
- Industrial pollutants
- Petrochemical fuels
- Pigments
- Paint and dyes
- Perfumes
- Preservatives
- Firsthand and secondhand pharmaceuticals—firsthand via prescriptions and over-the-counter pills; secondhand via residues in our water and animal-based food

The effects of these toxins can be difficult to trace and can vary from person to person. Toxins also interact with each other and with our bodies' own unique makeup in potentially harmful ways. The good news is, despite the toxic world we have, we still control most of what we allow into our bodies. This chapter will show you exactly how to weed out as many of these toxins as possible to reduce body burden using awareness and strategic lifestyle, nutrition, and supplementation choices.

DETOX—WHAT IT IS; HOW IT WORKS

Patients often come to me confused about "detoxing," because their doctors have told them there is no need to detoxify via cleansing or nutrition, because our bodies naturally detoxify themselves through the kidneys, liver, etc.

This is partially true; detoxification is an ongoing, natural process that occurs twenty-four hours a day, seven days a week, 365 days a year. *But,* our brilliantly designed bodies, though adaptable, were not made to process the sheer volume of toxins present in today's world. Therefore, I recommend all patients adopt specific detoxification strategies to optimize those burdened detox pathways.

Before we go on, let me clarify, when I say "specific detoxification strategies" this does not mean I expect you to isolate yourself from the world, avoid everything plastic, and fast or cleanse for weeks at a time—quite the opposite. The strategies I am about to share with you are incredibly practical and very easy to implement, so keep reading.

At its most basic level, detoxification works in two phases:[10]

- In Phase One, chemical reactions in the liver convert fat-soluble toxins into water-soluble toxins for easier elimination.
- In Phase Two, these are secreted into our urine or bile.

It is important to support both phases adequately, so your liver can do its work, and toxins can be excreted so they don't become a source of cell-damaging free radicals.

A little-known fact is the majority of detox takes place in the gut, with the rest of the gastrointestinal tract—lungs, kidneys, liver, and skin—playing important supporting roles.

Diets rich in antioxidants are naturally anti-inflammatory,[11] and therefore can decrease our vulnerability to chemical stressors. However, before you consider your first juice fast, keep in mind it is easy for detox to go wrong when embarked on too aggressively. Therefore, I recommend a gentle detox of the body burden first, before any extreme cleanses or fasts. With that in mind, let's discuss the best starting points and strategies for weeding out toxins.

WEEDING GUIDING PRINCIPLE 1: IMPROVE ELIMINATION

Improving elimination is listed first, as in doing so you will ensure the speedy removal of processed toxins and help facilitate a better balance of friendly, detoxifying gut bacteria. So, we must start with our poop!

The best ways to naturally improve elimination include:

- Staying hydrated—by consuming eight or more glasses of water a day—will help stimulate peristalsis (elimination) and keep everything flowing smoothly.
- Increasing your consumption of fruits and vegetables—for a natural source of fiber and gut-friendly prebiotics. Aim for two servings of fruit per day and ten to seventeen servings of vegetables.
- Trying the elimination diet—to simplify your diet and weed out any reactionary foods.
- Cutting out processed foods and refined sugars—these foods encourage an inflammatory state while robbing your body of essential nutrients.
- Practicing daily stress-relieving techniques—be mindful of the gut-brain connection and that fight or flight shuts down digestion. It's crucial to get serious about stress relief if you wish to improve elimination.
- Eating enough protein—will give your gut the building blocks it needs to repair and strengthen itself. Aim for a little over half (0.7 to be exact) of your body's weight in ounces per day.
- Eating your probiotics—though probiotic supplements make this easy, you can get amazing probiotic benefits from cultured foods like yogurt, kefir, kimchi, sauerkraut, and kombucha. Try eating them like a condiment by enjoying a little with every meal.

If you are following the advice from Chapter 3 on nourishment, you should already be seeing improvements in your elimination. If not, adopting some of these additional strategies will do the trick.

WEEDING GUIDING PRINCIPLE #2: GO ORGANIC...OR *MOSTLY* ORGANIC

Your second step in the weeding/detox process is to choose organic and naturally grown foods as much as possible. The reason is simple: Many commercial pesticides used in conventionally grown or raised foods are carcinogenic, laced with heavy metals,[12] and are known endocrine disruptors.[13]

If financial or other circumstances limit your access to organic foods, I suggest aiming to avoid what are known as "the dirty dozen" non-organic fruits and vegetables, and instead focus on eating more of "the clean fifteen." This list is available free from the Environmental Working Group, and is updated annually.

THE 2017 DIRTY DOZEN (PLUS THREE)

- Strawberries
- Spinach
- Nectarines
- Apples
- Peaches

- Pears

- Cherries

- Grapes

- Celery

- Tomatoes

- Sweet bell peppers

- Potatoes

- And the three extras: hot peppers, kale, and collard greens.

THE 2017 CLEAN 15

- Sweet corn

- Avocado

- Pineapple

- Cabbage

- Onions

- Frozen sweet peas

- Papayas

- Asparagus

- Mangoes

- Eggplant

- Honeydew

- Kiwi

- Cantaloupe

- Cauliflower

- Grapefruit

Don't forget about the wine! Organic wines are now widely available, close to sulfite-free (which means less headaches), and often cost less than conventional brands. Though I do not recommend drinking wine on the elimination diet, or if you have an autoimmune or hormonal condition, research, such as that published in the *New York Times'* best-selling book, *The Blue Zones* by Dan Buettner,[14] have shown its beneficial effects in relieving stress and increasing longevity. So, if you're going to have a drink, why not make it a clean and antioxidant-rich one?

The growing demand for organics has made them more affordable than ever, which is good news for everyone. You can save even more money by shopping your local farmer's market for a wide selection of certified-organic and naturally grown products,* signing up for a community supported agriculture (CSA) box program, and shopping price clubs (I list my favorite price clubs for organics in the resources section).

*Certified naturally grown products, usually found at farmer's markets, are certified by a peer-to-peer program, whereby farmer-members inspect each other's farms to ensure the food products they are selling are free from pesticides, herbicides, and other toxins. Think of "certified naturally grown" as the "organic" of the small farming industry.

Did you know, as of this writing in 2017, Costco Wholesale® (not Whole Foods Market®) is the #1 supplier of organics in the United States?

Regardless of the choices you make, it is important to invest in yourself and in your health, and nourishing yourself with organic, naturally grown foods as much as possible is one of the best ways to do this.

WEEDING GUIDING PRINCIPLE #3: DRINK AMAZING WATER

The third step is often overlooked by even the health-conscious crowd: Drink the purest and cleanest water possible. Besides the fact our bodies are 70 to 80 percent water, water also plays a crucial role in flushing toxins, maintaining blood volume, supporting skin elasticity and tone, and optimizing digestion.

Which water is best? Ideally, we would all be drinking natural spring water fresh from the source. Unfortunately, most of the spring water available today comes in plastic bottles that leach endocrine-disrupting chemicals like BPA and BPS. This leaves us with tap water, which is sanitary compared to the rest of the world—but the average city water supply is tainted with over 300 pollutants,[15] including heavy metals, pesticides, herbicides, raw sewage, mineral oil, gasoline, PCP, and pharmaceuticals.

Heavy metals found in water (and elsewhere) are of particular concern because of their cumulative effect on the nervous system and brain. Typically, the metals you see in public water are lead, arsenic, mercury, copper, and cadmium.[16] Fluoride, officially declared a neurotoxin by *The Lancet*,[17] is another chemical I recommend removing from your water.

According to the EPA, pharmaceuticals and personal care products have become "contaminants of emerging concern."[18] In 2010, scientists from the Southern Nevada Water Authority and other organizations reported results from a study analyzing drinking water from nineteen treatment plants. Their tests found antidepressants, antipsychotics, antibiotics, beta blockers, and tranquilizers, although only in trace amounts and far below levels, are thought to have an effect on humans.[19] Though many experts warn of a cumulative effect compounded by drinking eight (or more) glasses of contaminated water per day.

Well water is usually a safer choice than tap or bottled, but you need to have it tested for heavy metals (prevalent in pesticides and agricultural runoff), pesticides, bacteria, and mineral content to ensure you're getting a pure product. If you're unsure, it is best to filter your well water.

For most of us, use of a heavy-duty water filter is our best solution for pure, clean water. In choosing a water filter, it is important to go beyond the basics of chlorine and lead removal and seek out a filter that removes heavy metals, pharmaceuticals, viruses, fluoride, pesticides, and other endocrine disruptors. Reverse osmosis filters do the job well (though they strip out all the trace minerals from your water), as do specific carbon filtration systems, and other hybrid-models. The Environmental Working Group has an excellent tool to help you select the best filter for your needs and budget. See the resources section at the end of the chapter for more information on water filter recommendations.

One final thought on water: We need to be mindful about *reusable* water bottles. Again, plastic bottles, even BPA-free brands, will leach endocrine-disrupting chemicals into your beverages. Therefore, I recommend choosing either reusable stainless steel or glass bottles (see resources for more info).

WEEDING GUIDING PRINCIPLE #4: CONSUME DETOXIFYING FOODS AND SUPPLEMENTS

Your fourth step goes a little deeper to harness the power of detoxifying foods and professional-grade supplements.

Detoxifying foods will support Phase One and Phase Two detox while nourishing your elimination pathways and organs such as your liver, lungs, lymphatic system, gall bladder, skin, colon, urinary tract system, etc. See sidebar for recommendations.

PURIFYING PLANTS: THE TOP TEN FRUITS AND VEGETABLES FOR DETOX

- Brassica vegetables (broccoli, cauliflower, Brussels sprouts, etc.)
- Garlic
- Cherries
- Apples
- Raspberries
- Kelp and seaweed
- Chlorella
- Watercress
- Cilantro
- Pomegranates
- Allium family plants (onions, scallions, etc.)
- Lemon

DR. ALEX'S TWO-INGREDIENT DAILY DETOX TONIC:

This simple, inexpensive tonic is the essence of food as medicine. I recommend taking it upon rising, before bed, or any time your digestion feels off or sluggish.

1. Mix the juice of one fresh lemon with eight ounces of warm water. Add a little stevia, if desired, for sweetness.

2. Drink and enjoy either first thing in the morning or before retiring at night.

Lemons contain d-limonene, which has been shown to activate liver enzymes that are part of the Phase One and Phase Two detoxification processes. This tonic also helps stimulate peristalsis (elimination), and gently squeezes the gall bladder to keep fats and bile from building up.

Specific dietary supplements can be safely used to accelerate detoxification and support production of glutathione—your body's smart and protective antioxidant.

Examples of supplements that support detoxification include:

- Alpha lipoic acid
- B vitamins—specifically methylcobalamin and methylfolate.
- Dandelion
- Bitters
- Glutathione
- Green tea
- Magnesium
- Milk thistle
- NAC (N-acetyl-L-cysteine)
- Omega 3 fatty acids
- Probiotics
- Turmeric and curcumin
- Vitamin D3/K2

HEAVY METALS IN YOUR FOOD

Heavy metals are one of the sneakiest contributors to body burden, with many of them found in our food[10,11] and water.[13] When it comes to food, fish and seafood are of greatest concern. Though these foods have tremendous health benefits, many species have been tainted by heavy metals from industrial pollution of our waterways.

The Environmental Working Group recommends safe consumption of the following low-mercury fish:[20]

- Wild Alaskan salmon
- Pacific sardines
- Rainbow trout
- Atlantic mackerel
- Oysters
- Anchovies
- Pollock (imitation crab)
- Herring
- Shrimp
- Tilapia (from Ecuador or the United States)
- Scallops
- Clams
- Mussels

Conversely, avoid the following fish, which tend to be high in mercury:

- Canned light and albacore tuna
- Shark
- Swordfish
- Tilefish
- King mackerel
- Marlin
- Bluefin and bigeye tuna steaks or sushi
- Orange roughy
- Halibut
- Sea bass

Safe Catch® is an excellent seafood company to consider. They biopsy every single fish, and if it is high in mercury, they won't accept it. The Monterey Bay Aquarium's Seafood Watch program, www.seafoodwatch. org, also has ratings of the safety of different types of fish and seafood.

WEEDING GUIDING PRINCIPLE #5: RETHINK MAKEUP AND PERSONAL CARE PRODUCTS

While this might seem like a frivolous place to cut toxins, cosmetics and personal care products are a significant source of toxins for two reasons:

1. They are highly unregulated by the FDA.
2. We "ingest" them every single day via our skin, hair, teeth, nails, and lungs.

For example, cosmetic ingredients, such as parabens, are hormone disruptors;[21] common hair dyes and makeup products, such as lipsticks, often contain heavy metals;[22] studies have found health problems in people exposed to common fragrances;[23] and popular sunscreen ingredients carry a risk of sperm and reproductive system damage,[24] while countless other ingredients are known carcinogens.

According to the Environmental Working Group and other industry watchdogs, the FDA has no authority to require companies to test cosmetics for safety, and there are very few prohibited substances in cosmetics in the United States as compared to other Western countries.

The good news is, there is a whole wide world of non-toxic, natural, plant-based cosmetics, hair care (even hair color), and personal hygiene products out there for every style, budget, and taste. The EWG has created a database where you can find the cleanest sources of makeup and personal care products, and I have included a list of my personal favorite products in the resources section of this chapter.

DETOXING THE VAGINA

Feminine hygiene products are another prime point of entry for toxins. The skin around the vagina and the membranes within are very vulnerable and absorbent areas of the body.

Many feminine hygiene products have been bleached to get that pristine white color and contain chemically based odor neutralizers and fragrances. Chlorine is the most commonly used bleaching agent, and it can create disturbing side effects on its own—to say nothing of the pesticides used on the cotton grown to make these products. Furthermore, conventional sanitary pads contain plastic, which houses endocrine-disrupting chemicals like BPA and BPS.

Considering the tens of thousands of pads and tampons the average American woman uses in her lifetime, that's a whole lot of chemicals going straight into our reproductive systems.

Safer alternatives include:

- THINX® underwear

- 100% organic, chlorine-free tampons and pads.

- The DivaCup™.

- Reusable cotton pads.

See the resources section for links and more info.

Household cleaners are a HUGE source of unregulated, poisonous chemicals and toxins implicated in a slew of frightening diseases. This small sample of research proves my point:

- At least one study published in the *American Journal of Respiratory and Critical Care Medicine*[25] showed worsening symptoms in asthmatic women after completing household tasks, linking the worsened symptoms to conventional household cleaning products.
- Extensive studies show clear links between on-the-job exposure to cleaning supplies and the development of asthma in workers who have never shown previous signs of the disease.[26]
- Conventional cleaning products have also been linked to diseases as dramatic as cancer. Formaldehyde is a known human carcinogen, but is still an ingredient in many cleaners. 1,4-dioxane is also classified as a "likely human carcinogen" by the EPA,[27] but is still used in cleaning and skin care products.[28]
- A retrospective study by the Silent Spring Institute surveyed 1,500 Massachusetts women, half of whom had been diagnosed with breast cancer. The study suggested a link between using household cleaners and cancer, because the top 25 percent of women who reported high use of cleaning products were twice as likely to have been diagnosed with breast cancer as those reporting the least use.[29]

- Fragrances used in household cleaning products are collectively considered among the top five allergens in the world, and air fresheners in the home have been linked to higher incidences of diarrhea and earaches in infants and depression in their mothers.[30]
- A Swiss study found that the use of air freshening sprays four to seven days a week is associated with reduced heart rate variability,[31] a marker of autonomic dysfunction that increases sympathetic nervous system drive.

Despite these serious health concerns, the cleaning product industry is not required to label their products in a way that gives consumers the ingredient information they need to make informed choices.

LILY'S STORY

When I met Lily, she had already tried a lot of different things to improve her chronic fatigue syndrome. She had changed her diet to a degree, and while we adjusted it a little more, the most impactful thing she did was change her household cleaners and personal care products.

She stopped using traditional chemical household cleaners and switched all her body care products and makeup to non-toxic and natural products. When she removed those things from her body and environment, she noticed her fatigue improved, and she didn't feel so chemically sensitive—a common trait in chronic fatigue patients.

Lily had seen many different doctors, and she had done some modified elimination diets before, but no one had ever assessed her full lifestyle, including the possible pro-inflammatory household and personal care toxins fueling her chronic fatigue. When we assessed those together, her quality of life dramatically improved.

Lily's story is a perfect example of what can happen when we become aware of all the foreseeable toxins in our lives. Because these are what cause inflammation, and inflammation is at the root of ALL chronic (and many acute) diseases.

Given all this safety data—plus the obvious risks of keeping poisonous substances around—the sensible thing to do is to choose non-toxic cleaning products.

A Short-List of Cheap and Effective Non-Toxic Cleaners:

- Plain white vinegar can be diluted with water and used to clean surfaces, floors, windows, and mirrors.
- Baking soda mixed with castile soap makes an excellent scouring solution.
- Rubbing alcohol cleans mirrors way better than the "blue stuff."
- Essential oils are ideal for cleaning and sanitizing due to their natural antimicrobial properties. The best oils for all-purpose cleaning include tea tree, thyme, lemon, lavender, peppermint, cinnamon, and orange.
- For those who prefer to buy premade cleaning products, I recommend using the EWG's list included in the resources section, as (unfortunately) you can't trust manufacturer's labels.

Beyond household cleaners, we need to "clean house" by

becoming aware of other common toxins lurking in our homes and household products, including:

- Flame retardants—often found in baby and children's sleepwear, electronics, motor vehicles, furniture, textiles, mattresses, carpeting, and other household products).
  - Polybrominated diphenyl ethers (or PBDEs) are a class of flame retardants linked to short attention spans and issues with fine motor coordination and cognition in school age children. They are also linked to decreased fertility, thyroid problems, and myriad other issues.[32] The EPA said there is growing evidence that PBDE chemicals bioaccumulate and are persistent in the environment.
  - There is evidence these chemicals may cause liver toxicity, thyroid toxicity, and neurodevelopmental toxicity.[33]
- Household dust is where indoor pollutants, such as PBDEs, settle. Therefore, I advise:
  - Frequent dusting (preferably using vacuum attachments).
  - Use of an air filter.
  - Removing any old furniture that's begun to break down.
  - Choosing non-toxic, green-built furniture made with leather, wool, or cotton whenever possible. Non-toxic upholstery filled with cotton or polyester tends to be safer than chemically treated foam found in many low-end home furnishings.
  - Choosing non-toxic carpets and flooring, such as carpets made with 100% wool, bamboo, and other natural

fibers, and eco-friendly, non-toxic wood flooring treated without formaldehyde, etc.

- Kitchen toxins—beyond food:
  - o It's a good rule of thumb to avoid having plastics near your food. If you go out to eat at a restaurant, see if they have paper boxes or paper containers, especially if you're taking away hot foods. When you get coffee out, take the lid off. Plastics are bad enough for you, but heat makes things even worse.
  - o Teflon may be convenient, but it's also inconveniently toxic and a suspected carcinogen. You're far better off using stainless steel, cast-iron, or ceramic pots and pans.
- Electromagnetic fields (EMFs)—are the low-grade electrical fields produced by electronics—specifically cell phones, computers, and tablets. The World Health Organization, in 2011, classified EMFs from cell phones as possibly carcinogenic,[34] and other research has found connections between EMFs and lowered sperm counts,[35] a change in brain physiology,[36] and possible damage to unborn babies.[37]

Here's how to reduce your EMF exposure without going off-grid:

- Keep cellphones away from your head by using a speaker or hands-free device.
- Avoid using your phone when it has a weak signal as this increases EMF output.

- Use EMF-reducing tools like the DefenderPad® under your laptop, and radiation-reducing cell phone cases (see resources section).

- Keep your phone out of your bedroom and buy an alarm clock. Even on airplane mode, you don't want to sleep with a device near your head.

- Keep your children's screen time to a minimum. Their developing brains and bodies are much more susceptive to EMFs than are adults.

WANT TO FEEL HEALTHIER? ADOPT A NO-SHOE POLICY INDOORS

Shoes pick up all kinds of things, including pesticides, fertilizers, bacteria, fecal matter, and industrial pollutants, all of which are carried into your home, where they become sources of repeated exposure.

Taking off your shoes inside has been shown to lead to a significant reduction in lead, dust, and other chemicals, than were removed by using a doormat alone,[38] and it also decreases the bacteria you carry in to your house from, let's say a public restroom or sidewalk, removing the potential for infection from bacteria and viruses.

Weed your indoor garden of these sneaky toxins, and you will feel (and breathe) a lot easier.

The ABCs of Cleaning House:

1. Adopt a no-shoe policy.

2. Banish (or reduce exposure to) other indoor toxins such as flame retardants, dust, and kitchen toxins.

3. Choose non-toxic cleaners (or make your own).

Sweating and exercise play key roles in detoxification. Sweating alone has been shown to help rid the body of numerous toxins, including flame retardants,[39] BPA,[40] and heavy metals,[41]—yet most of us don't sweat nearly enough. For detox purposes, I recommend finding a way to sweat every single day.

Here are some easy ways to get your sweat on:

- Exercise—interval training, hot yoga, jogging, walking, circuit training, strength training, dancing, hiking, or any type of exercise that gives you that dewy glow.
- Saunas and/or steam rooms—I am partial to infrared saunas as they are incredibly efficient at pulling out toxins. You can find these saunas at spas, some gyms, wellness centers, or you can buy your own at varying prices. See resources section for more info on at-home saunas.
- Epsom salt baths—not only make you hot and sweaty, but also provide your body with a good dose of magnesium—a mineral of which many are deficient.
- Steamy showers—for added detox benefits, try simulating the infamous "cold plunge" by switching your shower from hot to cold. This stimulates circulation to mobilize and eliminate more toxins (plus, it's great for your hair and skin).
- Rebounding—though this is a form of exercise, I mention it separately because the up and down motion coupled with the

enhanced G-force of rebounding is one of the most effective ways to increase circulation and help move your lymphatic system—one of your main detoxification pathways.

MEET YOUR LYMPHATIC SYSTEM— THE BODY'S DRAINAGE SYSTEM

The lymphatic system, a gigantic network of lymph nodes, fluid, organs, and blood vessels, is one of our main systems of detoxification.

This miraculous system flows from our necks to our feet, and is responsible for shuttling essential fluids throughout the body and protecting us from outside threats (like viruses, bacteria, toxins, etc.) by producing and transporting disease-fighting white blood cells called lymphocytes.

The lymphatic system functions much like the circulatory system, but it does not have an automated pump. Therefore, it relies on regular movement to keep its fluid flowing freely. This, I believe, is one of the main reasons our sedentary lifestyle makes us so tired; no or limited movement means poor lymphatic flow, which leads to lymphatic congestion, increased body burden, fatigue, greater susceptibility to viruses, skin issues (including cellulite), and congestion.

Here are some ways to improve lymphatic health for increased energy, immunity, and improved skin tone:

- Get regular exercise—brisk walking and rebounding are considered the best exercises for the lymphatic system.

- Dry skin brushing—using a natural bristle body brush, brush in firm, upward strokes toward your heart. Start at your feet and work your way up. The helps move your lymphatic fluid while improving skin tone and texture.

- Infrared saunas.

- Massage and foam rolling.

Of all the toxins discussed in this chapter, emotional toxins require the most diligence in weeding. Why? Emotions are at the root of chronic stress, and chronic stress leads to inflammation and body burden, which is at the root of ALL chronic disease.

Here are some tips on how to weed your emotional garden on a regular basis:

- Stop complaining—chronic complaining has become a plague of modern society, and it's so insidious most of us don't notice how often we default to complaining. The problem with complaining is, like any habit, it signals your brain to create new pathways, which makes future complaining a no-brainer. In other words, it rewires your brain to focus on negativity instead of gratitude. What's more, research from Stanford University has proven chronic complaining leads to brain damage and memory loss by shrinking your hippocampus.[42] The first steps to weeding complaining from your life are to become aware of it and take steps to reframe complaint-based statements into more positive statements. Gratitude journaling, focusing on an attitude of expansion, and surrounding yourself with positive people will go leaps and bounds toward helping you break the complaining habit.
- Stop trying to be perfect—the pursuit of perfection goes

back to your attitude and state of mind. A perfectionist attitude desires a fixed end result—a stagnant place, where you are in control and everything is just so. What's wrong with this picture? Well first off, nothing in life stays the same, so you're setting yourself up for failure. Plus, it leaves no room for growth, expansion, or adventure. What's more, a perfectionist attitude has been linked to eating disorders and increases your risk of anxiety and depression. These feelings often come to the surface in the form of negative self-talk or beating yourself up when you fail to live up to your own (or anyone else's) expectations. If you find yourself caught in that perfectionist state of mind, take steps to gently bring yourself back to an attitude of expansion through journaling, prayer, meditation, etc.

- Be mindful of fear—like the fight-or-flight response, fear is a natural reaction that helps us survive. However, fear can become toxic if it creeps into your everyday life. I often tell my patients to think about their thoughts like a radio station and ask themselves, "Is there a good station on or a not so good one?" If it's a not so good station, then calmly change the station without judgment or self-criticism. We all experience fearful thoughts: the key is to become aware of when they take over and adjust your station accordingly. Refraining from screens and media can go a long way, as will regular meditation, switching your attitude and state of mind, and re-evaluating who you spend your time and energy with. It *is* a scary and dangerous world out there, but it is a kind and beautiful one too. Which world do you want to live in and contribute to? Your thoughts become your reality—so choose them wisely.

DR. ALEX'S BEST EMOTIONAL DETOX TOOLS

Many of our emotional toxins can be weeded at home through personal work. However, if you find the same negative emotions recurring again and again, that is a signal it is time to get a little extra help.

This list of best emotional detox tools includes exercises you can do yourself and with a caring mental health professional:

- Meditation and practicing mindfulness—this will help you become an observer of your thoughts, making it easier to choose a non-toxic path. Apps like Headspace® are excellent for this, or you can join a meditation group.
- Hypnosis—many of our thoughts, beliefs, and emotions are tied to early childhood experiences within our subconscious. A good hypnotist can help you break through these old patterns and realize a new way of life. Hypnosis has worked miracles for many of my patients.
- Tapping—also known as the emotional freedom technique, or EFT, involves using your fingertips to tap on different energetic points of your body connected to specific emotions.

You can learn the basics for free and it is highly effective. See resources for more information.

- Cognitive behavioral therapy—is practiced with a professional therapist, and can be a wonderful way to help you re-pattern old habits, sleep better, and let go of emotional baggage that is holding you back.
- Taking time in your sacred space—here you can practice daily meditation, gratitude journaling, tapping, etc., which will help you weed your garden.

WEEDING WAYS

Incorporate detox practices into your own life as frequently as possible.

Take steps to reduce exposure to toxins in your home, your food, and your grooming habits.

Examine and try to discard toxic thoughts and beliefs.

Work smarter, not harder.

You have done tremendous work in Step 4 by beginning to weed toxins from your life. We have also covered a huge amount of information, and you may be feeling overwhelmed. If you are, I invite you to stop, take a breath, and start with the action steps outlined below. Above all, remember to be patient and compassionate with yourself and take it one step at a time. In the next chapter, we move onto Step 5, where we will discuss the important role of your gut microbiome in supporting the healthy growth of your seeds, including enhancing immunity, preventing autoimmune disease, quelling inflammation, and balancing emotions.

Weeding Action Items:

- Choose one goal to accomplish this week from the weeding guiding principles outlined:
  - Improve elimination
  - Go organic (or mostly organic)
  - Drink the BEST water
  - Consume detoxifying foods and supplements
  - Rethink makeup and personal care products
  - Clean house
  - Get ready to sweat
  - Weed Emotional toxins with reckless abandon

Then, next week, add another guiding principle, or two, or more, depending on how you feel.

- Click on the resource section links below for helpful tools to help you on your weeding journey.

WEED Resources at nourishmedicine.com/bloomresources:

- EWG's Water Filter Buying Guide

- EWG's Consumer's Guide to Seafood
- Info on where to get the safest fish and seafood
- EWG's Guide to Healthy Cleaning
- EWG's Skin Deep Cosmetic Database
- Links to Dr. Alex's favorite natural feminine hygiene products
- EMF-reducing tools
- Recommendations for at-home infrared saunas
- Learn emotional freedom technique (EFT) basics for FREE
- Dr. Alex's favorite skin care products and brands

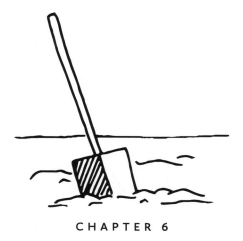

Step 5: ENRICH— The Gut

Up until this point, we have been focusing on the steps you must take to revitalize your existing state of health by rebuilding your strength and eliminating toxins. Now that you have a thorough understanding of those foundational steps, Step 5 will shift the focus to *preventative healing* through regular enrichment of your gut soil.

One of the golden rules of organic gardening and perma-culture is the more time you spend amending and caring for your soil, the less time you will spend on weeding and pest control. Step 5's guiding principles will teach you the little-known essentials of cultivating excellent gut health, including:

- What you need to know about women, stress, and the gut-brain connection.
- The causal factors behind gut imbalances.
- How to enrich your gut soil to sustain your seeds and blooms to prevent pests and toxins from taking over.

Please bear in mind, this chapter contains some of the most important information you will ever learn about preventing acute and chronic disease—therefore, I urge you to pay close attention to the details as we move through this vital step together.

A CRASH COURSE IN THE GUT MICROBIOME

In ancient Greece, the gut was viewed as the seedbed of good health, and recent research on the gut microbiome has confirmed that seedbed theory.

The microbiome is made up of a dizzying collection of trillions of bacteria, viruses, fungus, and other microbes that form the basis for immunity and protect us from unwanted invaders. The majority of these microbes are bacteria, and the largest populations reside in the gut. At present, science estimates there are as many microbial species in the body as there are human cells, with the average person harboring 30 trillion to 50 trillion microbes existing in symbiotic relationships. The actual number of bacterial microbes will vary from person to person, with women harboring more microbiota than men. Typically the microbiome approximates 0.3 percent of a person's total body weight.[1]

Our microbiome is established at birth, either through direct contact with vaginal secretions in the birth canal, and/or in a limited capacity via skin contact after birth. Those microbiota continue to diversify throughout our lifetime as we gain exposure to different environments, foods, germs, etc.

If that's not enough to blow your mind, consider this: Each person's gut microbiome is as unique as their fingerprint, and each of these unique microbes contains its own set of genes that influence how the body functions. Our gut microbiota and genome directly affect immune health, detoxification processes, emotional and mental well-being (via the enteric nervous system/gut-brain connection), behavior, digestion, metabolism, and nutrient processing.[2]

In other words, the gut is a big deal—far bigger than we thought just ten years ago. We are still in the infantile stages of understanding its vast influence on our physical, mental, and emotional health and our genetics.

Now, it's time to slip on our gardening gloves and dig a little deeper into how the miraculous world of the gut works, and why it tends to be such a hot bed of health issues for women.

WOMEN, STRESS, AND THE GUT-BRAIN CONNECTION

The gut-brain connection plays a crucial role in our ability to enrich and amend our gut soil. Yet, despite all the research, books, and buzz about "the second brain," very few people realize the detrimental effects of chronic stress on the gut.

Women are particularly vulnerable, because we tend to spend a lot of time in that fight-or-flight response: worrying, stressing, not sleeping, and taking care of everyone but ourselves. When we experience this level of chronic stress, it causes our bodies to release inflammatory stress hormones and immune system chemicals,[3] such as norepinephrine, cortisol, and cytokines—molecules that regulate immunity and inflammation. This forces the body into an inflammatory and immune-depressed state, causing your gut to become permeable and thus vulnerable to overgrowth of unfriendly yeast, bacteria, and pathogens,[4] while suppressing your gut's beneficial bacteria.[5]

INFLAMMATION—UNDERSTANDING THE ROOT CAUSE OF CHRONIC DISEASE

Inflammation is quickly being recognized as the leading causal factor behind many of the world's most chronic diseases, including heart disease, irritable bowel syndrome, allergies, autoimmune diseases, diabetes, inflammatory skin issues,[6] cancer,[7] and even depression and mental illness.[8]

Though these findings represent a huge stride for advancing medical treatment of these conditions, most experts still fail to ask the big question: *Why have we become so inflamed in the first place? What started the inflammatory process?*

The answer: One of the primary places inflammation begins is in the gut. Inflammation is initiated by a stress of some sort, be it emotional stress, a food sensitivity, or an environmental stressor like cigarette smoke or plastics. If that stressor is addressed quickly, then the inflammation goes away. However, if that stressor is not recognized and addressed promptly, that stressor will slowly wear down your immune system, resulting in a variety of unusual symptoms that progress from mild to severe over time. Since the gut makes up most of the immune system and is directly connected to the brain via the vagus nerve, which shuttles those stress hormones back and forth, it is the first system to become compromised by inflammation. This usually takes the form of leaky gut syndrome.

Being that the symptoms of leaky gut are so insidious, it is often overlooked allowing inflammation to spread throughout the body. This can result in more serious conditions such as chronic skin conditions, food sensitivities, and autoimmune disease.

Chronic inflammation is a mainstay of diabetes, cancer, autoimmune disease, and depression, to name a few, and they don't start overnight. Often, they are the result of a long-standing inflammatory response that began in the gut. The good news is, if we heal the gut using the principles and tools outlined in this chapter, the more serious conditions will naturally resolve in the process.

Unfortunately, it is a two-way street. Once you *have* leaky gut, it will then cause your brain more stress, which affects your digestion and immunity repeatedly. This may take the form of physical symptoms—like constipation or food sensitivities—or psychological problems—including depression,[9] anxiety, mood swings,[10] and panic attacks.[11]

This is why I have spent so much time emphasizing the importance of self-care within this book, because you cannot heal your gut (and reclaim your health, cultivate your desires, and reignite your spark) unless you are willing to address the underlying issue of chronic stress.

THE MYSTERIOUS SYMPTOMS OF A COMPROMISED GUT

The most difficult thing for patients with gut-health problems is not necessarily treating them (because they're not that hard to fix); it's finding a knowledgeable doctor who knows how to recognize their symptoms and diagnose them correctly. Roughly 80 percent of the patients I see wind up on my doorstep because their doctors were unable to connect the dots of their "random" symptoms to gut malfunction. This often leaves patients feeling sick, confused, and led to believe their symptoms must be "unrelated" or, worse, "all in their head," when nothing could be further from the truth.

The following is a list of common symptoms and conditions shown or observed in practice to be rooted in gut-health issues:

- Acid reflux
- Acne[12]
- Autoimmune disease[13]
- B12 deficiencies
- Dysbiosis
- Chronic congestion
- Depression, anxiety, mood swings[4,5]
- Diabetes[14]
- Eczema
- Fatigue/burnout
- Food sensitivities
- Fungal skin conditions such as athlete's foot
- Headaches[15]
- Irritable bowel syndrome[16]
- Psoriasis and other inflammatory skin issues[17]
- Thyroid issues
- Weight gain
- Yeast infections
  - Yeast overgrowth

As you can see, this list runs the gamut with many symptoms considered conditions in and of themselves. However, as we dig a little deeper using the functional medicine approach, we nearly always trace the symptoms and conditions back to a gut-related issue.

MAJOR CONTRIBUTORS TO POOR GUT HEALTH

Aside from chronic stress, there are numerous other foods, toxins, and lifestyle factors that disrupt gut microbiota balance, leading to a breach in the intestinal tract.

- Chronic stress[4]—had to mention it again.
- A diet high in processed foods,[18] particularly gluten[19,20,21]—this leads to nutrient deficiencies, increased inflammation, and causes an overgrowth of "bad" bacteria.
- Multiple-rounds of antibiotics kill your friendly bacteria, resulting in an overgrowth of "bad" bacteria.[22]
- History of food poisoning—this often weakens the digestive tract leaving you susceptible to leaky gut.
- Over-sanitization—though cleanliness is important, our modern, ultra-sterile foods, environments, and products have taken a toll on gut bacteria diversity.[23] See sidebar for more information.
- Regular use of NSAIDs—this quickly breaks down your intestinal wall.[24]
- History of steroid or corticosteroid use.

- Genetics—this is not true for everyone, but genetics, including genetic mutations, can play a role in gut health.[25]
- Nutrient deficiencies[26]—such as B12, iron, and zinc caused by poor diet, medications, and genetic mutations.
- C-section birth—new research has proven babies born by C-section have a less diversified gut microbiota than those born vaginally.[27] This is because they do not receive beneficial microbes that would have been transferred from their mother during their time in the birth canal. See sidebar "Healthy Tummies: Gut Health for Kids" for more information.

WANT A HEALTHIER GUT? EMBRACE THE DIRT

One of the easiest and most profound ways to improve your gut-health diversity and boost immunity is to spend more time outdoors. Direct contact with microbes found in the soil, floating through fresh air, in the trees, water, and even on farm animals and pets educates our immune system by forcing our bodies to fight off harmless bacteria. This results in greater gut microbiota diversity and a smarter immune system.

Studies have shown children who are regularly exposed to dirt and germs, on farms for example, and aren't overly sanitized have stronger immune systems and lower incidences of asthma and eczema.[18] Other studies, such as those conducted at Johns Hopkins, show that newborns exposed to dirt, dander, and germs may have a lowered risk of asthma and allergies.[28]

While hygiene is important, it's easy to overdo it with antibacterial soaps, hand sanitizers, synthetic antibacterial ointments, etc. Instead, opt for natural soaps and plant-based hand sanitizers. Bottom line, the more dirt and natural microbes to which children and adults are exposed, the healthier the gut and the stronger the immune system will be.

FUNCTIONAL MEDICINE'S APPROACH TO HEALING THE GUT

As you can see, the roots of gut imbalance and disease are complex and interwoven. Therefore, functional medicine takes a diverse approach to enriching and repairing the gut using a specific sequence of diet and lifestyle changes. In my practice, I typically follow this three-step gut healing system:

Gut-Health Guiding Principle #1: Eliminate Trigger Foods and STRESS

We start by using an elimination diet and/or lab tests to identify exactly which foods are irritating the gut. Common trigger foods include:

- Gluten
- Dairy
- Soy
- Eggs
- Grains (including corn)
- Sugar
- Alcohol
- Those with autoimmune conditions may also need to eliminate nuts, and nightshade vegetables (potatoes, tomatoes, peppers, and eggplant).

In addition, we use the steps discussed in Chapter 5: Weed and Chapter 4: Root to identify common stressors and prescribe self-care rituals and strategies to neutralize them. Specifics on lab work for detecting leaky gut are outlined in Chapter 7: Prune.

Gut-Health Guiding Principle #2: Amend and Enrich the Soil

Once we have identified and eliminated the trigger foods, we work on amending the gut soil with nutrients, and enriching the gut with friendly bacteria using specific foods and supplements.

Food and Supplement Amendments:

- Digestive enzymes—a compromised gut equals compromised digestion. Therefore, by supplementing with enzymes, we ensure food is broken down and utilized efficiently.
- Hydrochloric acid—for those with specific digestive issues, a natural HCL supplement can help relieve digestive stress.
- Apple cider vinegar, bitters, or lemon water before meals can help naturally increase your production of hydrochloric acid.
- Bone broth—rich in natural gelatin, collagen, amino acids, glutamine, glycine, and minerals, real bone broth soothes and nourishes your gut while providing the building blocks for cellular repair.
- Plenty of fruits and vegetables provide easy-to-digest vitamins,

minerals, enzymes, prebiotic fiber, and phytonutrients. Aim for ten to seventeen servings a day.

- Aloe vera juice soothes and coats irritated tissues while supporting normal elimination.
- Slippery elm bark has soothing and healing mucilage properties that support the gut mucosa.
- Marshmallow—this herb contains mucilage properties, eases inflammation, and helps protect the lining of the digestive system.
- L-Glutamine—an amino acid essential to gut repair and maintenance.
- Zinc gluconate (chelated) or zinc citrate, B12 (methylcobalamin)—compromised gut health often results in a vitamin B12 deficiency.[21] Zinc supplementation has been shown to support repair of the gut lining.[29]

Enriching Foods and Supplements:

Here, we enrich by re-inoculating the gut with friendly bacteria from foods and supplements.

- Cultured foods, such as yogurt, kimchi, kombucha, kefir, and sauerkraut, are brimming with naturally occurring probiotics and enzymes to re-seed the gut.
- Probiotic supplements—look for professional-grade multi-strain formulas with at least 50 CFUs, and no added sugar, preservative, or artificial colors or flavors.

In addition to its obvious gut-health benefits, probiotic supplementation has been shown to decrease the risk of upper respiratory tract infection in adults and in children.[30] There is also some correlation between microbiota and change in body composition, which indicates probiotics can influence energy metabolism in obesity.[31]

THE CRUCIAL ROLE OF PREBIOTICS IN PROBIOTIC THERAPY

Prebiotics are the natural indigestible fibers found in certain plants and act as a food source for probiotics to live on and proliferate. Without prebiotics, probiotics cannot survive and diversify in the gut.

Plant sources of prebiotics include:

- Onions
- Leeks
- Garlic
- Jicama
- Chicory
- Dandelion greens
- Jerusalem artichoke

Gut-Health Guiding Principle #3: Maintaining Gut Soil Health

Once the root causes have been resolved, and the gut is healed and enriched, the maintenance phase begins (and life gets a whole lot easier).

How to Maintain Healthy Gut Soil

- Keep your stress in check by practicing daily self-care rituals.
- Avoid your trigger foods.
- Continue eating plenty of fruits, vegetables, whole foods, and cultured foods.
- Enjoy bone broth one to three times a week.
- Avoid antibiotics whenever possible (see sidebar).
- Challenge and diversify your gut microbiome by spending plenty of time outdoors and avoiding antibacterial soaps and cleaning products.
- If you're over thirty years old, consider continuing digestive enzyme supplementation as our enzyme stores decrease with age.

NATURAL ALTERNATIVES FOR SUPPORTING IMMUNITY

Despite the fact that antibiotic resistant superbugs are killing over 700,000 people a year globally,[32] my experience in primary and urgent care taught me that we still rely on antibiotics far too heavily.

Antibiotics do have their place in certain situations, but we must take steps to educate ourselves on alternatives, if we are to have any hope of weathering this superbug crises and protecting our gut health and immunity.

Time-honored natural remedies traditionally used and/or shown to support immunity while protecting gut microbiota diversity include:

- Bone broth[33]
- Colloidal silver (applied in the ear, not taken internally please)
- Echinacea[34]
- Elderberry syrup[35]
- Essential oils of mint, cinnamon, thyme, clove, oregano,[36] and eucalyptus[37]
- Garlic[38]
- Garlic/mullein oil (applied in the ear or massaged into the feet)
- Ginger[39]
- Olive leaf[40]
- Oscillococcinum[41] (a homeopathic used and shown to prevent the onset and to shorten the duration of the flu)
- Probiotics[42]
- Turmeric/curcumin[43]
- Vitamin C[44]
- Vitamin D[45]
- Zinc lozenges[46]

As with any natural remedies, it is important you work with a qualified integrative health practitioner to determine appropriate dosing of these herbs and nutrients for you.

Remember, the most powerful way to avoid antibiotics and other gut-harming medications in the first place is to tend and enrich your gut soil regularly.

GUT FACTS[47]

- The gut produces three-quarters of the body's neurotransmitters.

- It contains at least two-thirds of the body's immune system.

- It houses the majority of your microbiome.

HEALTHY TUMMIES: GUT HEALTH FOR KIDS

The health and diversity of the microbiome starts at birth with the transfer of microbiota from mother to child in the birth canal. If a baby must be born C-section, many doctors and midwives now take swabs from the mother's vagina to spread on the baby's mouth and nose when the child is born. This allows the child to populate their own microbiome with the bacteria that would have been present in a vaginal birth.

After birth, breast milk takes over as baby's first microbiome-enriching, immune-boosting superfood. The number of beneficial bacteria, probiotics, prebiotics, and other nutrients in breast milk are *still* being discovered, and there is no question that it is truly nature's perfect food.

As a baby grows up, we can continue diversifying their microbiome through exposure to the great outdoors, playing in the dirt, not over-sanitizing them (within reason); encouraging a healthful diet with plenty of veggies and cultured foods, and avoiding antibiotics, steroids, NSAIDS, and antibacterial products whenever possible.

A healthy microbiome is one of the greatest gifts you can give to the next generation.

PSYCHOBIOTICS FOR MENTAL HEALTH AND PAIN

Researchers have discovered a group of probiotic bacteria specific to regulating mental health and reducing pain called psychobiotics. They work by reducing levels of the stress hormone, cortisol, and by working through the immune system to decrease inflammation,[48] now a recognized causal factor behind depression.

I have often witnessed when patients take the time to enrich their gut soil for physical reasons, like to clear up psoriasis or fix a digestive issue, they wind up mitigating their mood disorders at the same time (much to their delight).

WHEN TO SEEK HELP ENRICHING YOUR GUT SOIL

Though there is so much you can do yourself to enrich and diversify your gut microbiome, those with chronic gut-related inflammatory issues would be well-advised to partner with a functional medicine physician. A medical doctor experienced in integrative and functional medicine can order the right advanced diagnostic tests—such as stool tests and food sensitivity panels—to develop an individual treatment plan. For example, someone with an autoimmune condition will likely need different supplementation and dietary guidelines than someone with irritable bowel syndrome or migraines, and a good doctor will be able to advise you on the most effective therapies for your individual needs.

Now that you have fearlessly delved into the vast world of the gut microbiome and learned how to prevent disease through enrichment, you're ready to move onto Chapter 7,

Step 6: Prune. This step is all about getting "unstuck" from your current state of health with help from a functional medicine physician. We will discuss the most common underdiagnosed conditions most doctors miss; plus, everything you need to know about finding the right physician and healthcare team, and what types of advanced lab tests to ask for in the pruning process.

Enriching Action Items:

1. Ask yourself: Am I taking my self-care and stress management practices seriously? It will make or break your gut health. If you have skipped days or slacked in this area, it's time to recommit to daily practice.

2. Look at the list of gut-related symptoms in this chapter and put a checkmark next to any that apply to you. If your checkmarks relate to an acute or simple issue, use the principles outlined in this chapter; if it's a more chronic or complex issue, consider partnering with a functional medicine doctor for faster resolution (more on how to find one in the next chapter).

3. Review my 3 guiding principles for enriching your gut, and commit to adopting three new gut-enriching practices this week. For example, #1: I will spend at least thirty minutes outdoors, #2: I will eat probiotic-rich foods like kombucha and yogurt every day, and #3: I will replace my antibacterial soaps with natural soaps.

Write down what you will do in the spaces below:

Gut Soil Enriching Practice 1:

Gut Soil Enriching Practice 2:

Gut Soil Enriching Practice 3:

ENRICH Resources at nourishmedicine. com/bloomresources:

- Recommended apps for meditation
- Dr. Alex's favorite Premade Bone Broth
- Dr. Alex's favorite gut-health products

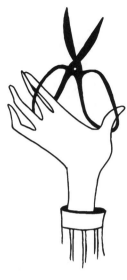

CHAPTER 7

Step 6: PRUNE— Getting Unstuck

———

At this point in the journey, we have thoroughly prepared your garden to Bloom. We have prepped the soil by cultivating an attitude of expansion, carefully selected your seeds of desire and planted them in the nourished soil of intention. We have nurtured a strong root system through self-care practices and begun the process of identifying and eliminating toxic weeds and enriching your gut soil. Our sixth step in this chapter is to prune.

For those who haven't attempted it, pruning a tree or plant takes special skills and knowledge—prune at the wrong time of year and you will shock or damage your plants; prune too little or in the wrong place and you can stunt growth. The same principle applies to your Bloom process, which is why, at this stage, you may benefit from some professional advice. Specifically, if you are at a point where you have made significant changes, yet still can't quite reignite that "spark" of energy or are stuck with the same old unwanted symptoms, you could be experiencing *deficiencies* or a *subclinical condition* that requires lab work ordered by a physician.

This chapter will help you understand *if* you have the type of deficiencies that require a professional pruner aka functional medicine physician, PLUS, we will cover everything you need to know about finding the right doctor and health-care team to help you reach full Bloom faster.

WHEN YOU *FEEL* LIKE YOU'RE DOING EVERYTHING RIGHT BUT YOU STILL DON'T *FEEL* RIGHT

The best indicator of when to seek professional help is when you have already made conscious shifts in your diet, lifestyle, and environment yet still don't feel quite right.

Kelly's story is a perfect example of a patient who had done everything she could on her own to improve her health, yet she still suffered a myriad of puzzling symptoms.

When Kelly came to see me, she was already on top of her nutrition and had a firm grasp on many natural living principles. However, despite her healthy lifestyle, she was still suffering from weight gain, poor digestion, embarrassing bloating, sluggishness, and fatigue. She had been to her family doctor, yet her labs had all come back "normal," so she sought me out. As part of my normal intake process, I ran a series of advanced lab tests on her. When the results came back, we discovered she had a host of issues we would not have found otherwise.

She had severe iron-deficiency anemia, vitamin D deficiency, fungal overgrowth in her gut, low vitamin B12, and an underactive thyroid. No wonder she was feeling so poorly! We then tested her for food sensitivities and found she was highly reactive to dairy. As if all that weren't enough, she was also pre-diabetic.

Many of my patients are in the same predicament as Kelly, with multiple problems all impacting each other. In Kelly's case, her iron-deficiency anemia was hampering her body's ability to make thyroid hormone; her vitamin D deficiency left her vulnerable to multiple infections, which also kept her body from making thyroid hormone efficiently; her B12 deficiency meant she couldn't make red blood cells, which impacted her iron levels, leaving her feeling fatigued; and the fungal overgrowth in her gut exacerbated all these nutrient deficiencies, leaving her body unable to fully heal.

With Kelly, we set goals, then got right to work, enriching her gut and correcting the micronutrient deficiencies causing this cascade effect. Within a short time, she got her energy back, then her thyroid symptoms reversed, because she had the nutrients she needed. Based on her food sensitivity panels, we changed her diet by removing dairy, grains, alcohol, and sugar, and this reversed her pre-diabetes and the fungal overgrowth. Within a four-month period, she was no longer anemic, her vitamin D levels reached optimal range, her gut was healed, and her blood sugar and thyroid function have improved dramatically.

Kelly's case is, in many ways, typical. She was trying to push through when she didn't feel well. When things got bad, she sought medical attention only to be dismissed with "normal" lab results. She also didn't realize how bad she felt until she began to feel *normal* again.

It has been said, "You can't master what you don't measure," and a trained functional medicine physician will have the advanced labs, intake skills, and other technologies to measure these fundamental aspects of health. Without this vital information, how would a person know exactly what to prune?

WHAT TO DO WHEN "YOUR LABS ARE NORMAL," BUT YOU DON'T FEEL WELL?

Many of my patients, like Kelly, wind up feeling desperate to find a solution when their providers tell them, "Your lab work is normal; there's nothing wrong with you."

On an intuitive level, no one knows your body better than you do. If you know something is wrong, something is probably wrong, and you must keep looking for a provider who is willing to sit down, listen, and go those extra miles to figure it out with you.

NUTRIENT DEFICIENCIES: THE MOST COMMON UNDERDIAGNOSED HEALTH ISSUE IN WOMEN

Before we go through the how-tos on finding and assembling your star team of healthcare providers, I want to run through this list of the most common underdiagnosed health issues I see in women, which are often at the root of many diseases.

As discussed in Chapter 3: Nourish, food provides

information in the form of nutrients that our bodies need to function optimally. If we aren't getting enough nutrients from our diet, our health will suffer. Beyond diet, other factors can influence our ability to absorb, assimilate, and utilize nutrients from our food, such as:

- Depleted topsoil—over the last half-century our topsoil has been depleted of key nutrients which has degraded the nutrient quality of our food.[1] This means the fruits and vegetables we consume today are less nutrient-dense than they were fifty or one hundred years ago.[2]
- Compromised digestion—if your digestive system is off, due to leaky gut, insufficient enzymes, or consumption of certain medications, you cannot fully assimilate the nutrients you take in[3]
- Heavily processed and modified foods—processed foods, even organic ones, are not nutrient-dense and often contain heavily processed corn. In the United States, there is a direct link between large-scale production of corn and micronutrient deficiency.[4]
- A lack of traditional food preparation—as discussed in Chapter 3: Nourish, traditional cooking methods, such as fermenting bread before baking, were used to help break down anti-nutrients like phytic acid, while increasing the availability of key vitamins and minerals. Modern food preparation has streamlined things, but made food less nutritious and less digestible in the process.

This section will cover the top three nutrient deficiencies I see in most of my female patients, their lesser-known causes and symptoms, the lab tests you must ask for to root them out, and how to rebuild your nutrient stores naturally.

1. Iron deficiency

The World Health Organization estimates up to 42 percent of non-pregnant women and up to 52 percent of pregnant women have an iron deficiency known as anemia.[5]

Iron deficiency, even a mild deficiency, can cause a cascade of health issues as iron participates in a slew of bodily functions—from oxygen transport to making DNA. Iron is also essential for healthy blood that carries oxygen from our lungs throughout the body,[6] hence, why those with anemia are prone to fainting. Women are especially vulnerable to iron deficiency because, though iron is highly conserved by the body, much is lost during menstruation, and excessive menstrual blood loss is one of the most common cause of anemia in women.[7]

Here is where nutrient deficiencies like this get missed at the typical doctor's office: The official diagnosis of "anemia" refers to specific lab values, *but* you can still have an iron deficiency that is not classified as "anemia." This is where most lab tests fail the patient, because even mild or moderate forms of iron deficiency can be associated with functional impairments affecting cognitive development, morbidity (not feeling well overall), immunity mechanisms,[8] and your functional capacity to complete daily tasks.[9]

Lesser-Known Causes of Iron Deficiency (beyond excessive menstruation or blood loss):

- Impaired gastric acid production[10]—often due to proton pump inhibitors and antacids.
- Insufficient amounts of hydrochloric acid[11]—as discussed in the previous chapter, hydrochloric acid helps with nutrient absorption.
- Too much phytic acid in the diet[12]—found in grains and beans that can inhibit iron absorption.
- Genetic predispositions[13]—people of specific cultural backgrounds may be more prone to certain types of anemia than are others.
- Not enough iron in the diet—vegans and vegetarians especially often consume a lot of phytic-acid-rich foods like grains and legumes, while neglecting to eat enough iron-rich foods, putting them at greater risk for anemia.

SYMPTOMS OF IRON DEFICIENCY VS. FULL-BLOWN ANEMIA

Symptoms of Full-Blown Anemia:

- Fatigue

- Weakness

- Shortness of breath

- Headaches

- Fast heartbeat

- Cold hands and feet

- Lightheadedness and dizziness

- Fainting

Symptoms of Mild to Moderate Iron Deficiency:

- Fatigue

- Cognitive issues

- Lowered immunity

- Learning disabilities (mild to moderate)

- Not feeling well overall

Labs to Ask for If You Suspect Iron Deficiency:[14]

- CBC, with a hemoglobin less than 12
- An MCV less than 85
- Ferritin less than 30
- Serum ferritin is the best single laboratory test to diagnose iron deficiency.

Typically, physicians only check the CBC, see that everything is in the normal range, and don't bother to look at ferritin or transferrin saturation, which gives the full picture before full-blown anemia sets in. By gaining insight from just two other labs, you can often avoid anemia and resulting issues by changing your diet and/or supplementation.

Dr. Alex's Tips for How to Build Up and Enhance Iron Absorption:

- Increasing your vitamin C intake enhances your ability to absorb iron.[15]
- Getting enough heme-based iron from animal sources such as meat, poultry, and fish.[16]
  - Non-heme-based iron comes from plants and fruits and is less absorbable than heme.
- Supplement with a professional-grade iron supplement—buyer beware: lesser-quality supplements can be hard on your elimination and digestive system.
- Talk to your practitioner about a hydrochloric acid supplement.
- Chew your food thoroughly to support digestive enzyme production.
- Use cast-iron cookware.[17]
- If you have heavy periods, talk to your doctor about treatment options.

Have your labs re-checked after six weeks and discuss the need for any future treatment with your doctor.

2. Vitamin B12 Deficiency

Vitamin B12 deficiency results from an inability to absorb B12 in the small intestine[18] or from a lack of animal foods in the diet. Like iron deficiency, a lack of B12 means your body cannot make red blood cells correctly. B12 deficiency is a lot more common than most people realize, but it is most common in vegetarians and vegans[19] and in adults over the age of fifty—because our ability to absorb B12 reduces with age. It is estimated that 40 percent of adults over the age of sixty are B12 deficient in the "low-normal" range, with their B12-deficiency symptoms often masquerading as more serious cognitive and memory conditions.[20] You can also have a B12 deficiency that produces some unwanted symptoms but does not create pernicious anemia.

The Lesser-Known Causes of B12 Deficiency:

- Abnormal bacteria growth in the small intestine—also known as SIBO.[21]
- Inflammatory gut-health issues—such as inflammatory bowel disease or Crohn's Disease.[13]

- Intestinal parasites—rare, but not unheard of, especially for those who travel internationally.[22]
- Lack of "intrinsic factor" often caused by autoimmune disease[23]—intrinsic factor is a protein excreted by the stomach that allows B12 to be absorbed into the bloodstream. If you don't have the intrinsic factor, you can't absorb the B12 you're taking in. There is also an autoimmune disease, where your body attacks the parietal cells, which make intrinsic factor.
- Prescription medications—many patients are not aware that these medications deplete B12 stores
  - Azithromycin
  - Birth control pills
  - Cimetidine
  - Ciprofloxacin
  - Lansoprazole
  - Levaquin
  - Metformin
  - Minocycline
  - Omeprazole
  - Ranitidine

WHY IS VITAMIN B12 SO IMPORTANT?

Vitamin B12 works with folate, another B vitamin, to synthesize DNA and to make red blood cells. They also make the myelin sheath, which is the insulation around nerves. Your body is constantly trying to repair its DNA, and to do that, you need to be able to carry out a process called *methylation*.

Methyl folate and methyl B12 are used by the body to repair DNA; if your body can't add methyl groups to B vitamins, not only can it not repair DNA, it also cannot repair your immune system or make red blood cells. Inability to methylate is linked to a genetic deficiency.[24]

Symptoms of B12 Deficiency:

- Memory problems
- Tingling in hands and feet
- Fatigue
- Cognitive issues
- Difficulty walking
- A swollen, red tongue
- Paranoia or hallucinations
- Anemia

Labs to Ask For If You Suspect Vitamin B12 Deficiency:

- CBC (and your MCV is going to be high)
- A methylmalonic acid test
- Check your homocysteine, to determine whether you can properly methylate B12 and folate
- MTHFR genetic mutation testing—to determine if you have the MTHFR genetic mutation or variation of which affects your ability to methylate and utilize B12.
- Stool testing—for inflammatory intestinal issues
- Food sensitivity testing—may or may not be indicated based on your gut health

By American standards, B12 levels of less than 350 are

considered "low-normal," but even at 500, we can see psychological symptoms and cognitive decline. In my practice, I aim to keep patients closer to 1000 for optimal health benefits; keep this in mind when you receive your lab results.

Dr. Alex's Tips for How to Rebuild Vitamin B12 Stores:

- Supplement with methylcobalamin—an activated form of vitamin B12, sold in a lozenge form, that can be readily absorbed into your bloodstream even if you cannot methylate properly.
- Eat plenty of animal foods—red meats, liver, shellfish, and eggs are all excellent sources.
- Work on your gut health—as bacterial overgrowth and inflammatory issues are causal factors.
- Discuss possible alternatives to B12-depleted medications with your doctor.
- Have your doctor re-check your levels every eight weeks.

THE BASICS ON METHYLATION AND MTHFR GENETIC MUTATIONS:

It is estimated that millions of Americans have a variation of the MTHFR genetic mutation, which affects our methylation processes. Methylation is used in hundreds of different biochemical processes—not just repairing DNA, but also making neurotransmitters, cell repair, and supporting the immune system, among others.[25] When you have B-vitamin deficiencies due to poor methylation, you will have poor neurological healing, mitochondrial weakness, immune system issues, and poor toxin clearance. If you're not methylating well, you're not fixing things well. The whole idea with B12 and methylfolate supplementation is to hack that system and to help get the nutrients in so they are already methylated.

3. Vitamin D Deficiency

Despite increased awareness in the medical world, vitamin D deficiency is still a growing epidemic in women and men alike, for one big reason and one smaller reason:

- The big reason: We simply do not get enough sunlight.
- The smaller, lesser-known reason: Certain medications like statins and corticosteroids deplete what little vitamin D stores we have.

For years, we have been told to stay out of the sun or to use sunscreen outdoors; unfortunately, this, along with our indoor lifestyles, has caught up with us and widespread vitamin D deficiency is the result.

With this new understanding, experts are now recommending between fifteen minutes to two hours of unprotected sun exposure daily (depending upon your skin type). Doctors now also check patients' vitamin D levels regularly and often recommend high-dose supplementation. Unfortunately for us, many doctors are prescribing the wrong type of vitamin D supplement. It is now widely recognized that vitamin D3 is superior to vitamin D2; however, the synergistic relationship between vitamin D3 and vitamin K2 is still widely undervalued. If these two vitamins are not taken in combination, poor absorption and calcium-related health issues can result.

This is how vitamins D3 and K2 work together: When you take vitamin D, your body becomes more receptive to absorbing calcium. This is good thing, except you want that calcium going straight to your skeleton and away from your arteries, where it can create hardening over time. That's where vitamin K2 comes in—acting as a protective shuttle to move vitamin D and calcium to your bones and appropriate systems for absorption, while keeping calcium out of your arteries. Bottom line: Without proper amounts of vitamin K2, vitamin D and calcium won't be absorbed properly.

Symptoms of Vitamin D Deficiency:

- Arthritis[26]

- Autoimmune disease[27]
- Certain cancers[22]
- Chronic pain[22]
- Depression[22]
- Diabetes[22]
- Eczema[21]
- Fibromyalgia[22]
- Gut-health issues[21]
- Heart disease[21]
- Hormonal imbalance[21]
- Infertility[21]
- Insomnia[21]
- Lowered immunity[22]
- Metabolic issues including insulin resistance/pre-diabetes[22]
- Osteoporosis[22]

Lab Test to Ask for If You Suspect Vitamin D Deficiency:

- Have your doctor specifically order the test for 25-hydroxy vitamin D, also known as the 25-OH D test.
- The optimal amount is 45 to 65 ng/ml, and in some cases, even higher levels are appropriate.

Dr. Alex's Tips for How to Replenish and Maintain Healthy Vitamin D Levels:

The amount of vitamin D you will need to replenish deficiencies depends on your lab tests, so check with your provider for recommendations.

- Get enough unfiltered, unprotected sunlight a day (see sidebar and resources for recommendations).[28]
- If you need to supplement, choose a vitamin D3 supplement with vitamin K2, and work closely with your doctor to monitor your levels for safety reasons.
- Whole foods sources of vitamin D include shiitake and button mushrooms (leave them in the sun to elevate their vitamin D levels), mackerel, sockeye salmon, cod liver oil, sardines, and eggs.[22]

HOW MUCH SUN EXPOSURE IS SAFE FOR YOU?

This is a not a one-size-fits-all answer because of various factors, including:

- Your location
- The time of year
- The time of day
- Your skin type
- Your age
- The amount of skin you expose
- Your altitude
- And how sunny or cloudy it is on a given day

In addition, different experts and organizations recommend different amounts of daily vitamin D. For example, The Food and Nutrition Board recommends just 600 IUs for adults and 800 IUs daily for seniors, while the Vitamin D Council recommends 5000 IUs a day for adults.[29] In my experience and based on the current research, it pays to a moderate when it comes to sun exposure. Therefore, I recommend getting some unprotected sun exposure every day per the Vitamin D Council's recommendations for your skin type, location, etc. (see below), and protecting yourself with a non-toxic sunscreen once you have gotten your daily sun exposure.

According to The Vitamin D Council:[24]

- Those with very light to light skin likely need ten to fifteen minutes of unprotected sun exposure.
- Those with naturally tan skin can take unprotected sun for fifteen to twenty minutes.
- Those with darker skin can safely take one to two hours of unprotected sun exposure.

The key is not to let your skin burn. For those concerned about cancer, research has proven that a healthy amount of sun exposure can actually protect you from several types of cancer.[30] Again, do not overdo it.

See the resources section for more information on all the amazing protective health benefits of sunshine for adults and children.

WHAT ELSE COULD IT BE? THE TOP SEVEN UNDERDIAGNOSED CLINICAL AND SUBCLINICAL CONDITIONS PLAGUING MODERN WOMEN

Nutrient deficiencies aren't the only reason you could be feeling poorly. Oftentimes, as you've read about in the patient stories throughout the book, people come to me with "normal labs" feeling awful only to find out they were suffering from a very real condition. The following are the top clinical and subclinical conditions I can help patients discover using the integrative functional medicine approach and advanced lab work:

1. Hashimoto's Disease and Hypothyroidism

Hashimoto's Disease, an autoimmune condition where healthy cells attack the thyroid gland,[31] is extremely common in women and, sadly, often not diagnosed until it's late-stage.

Symptoms often include fatigue, thinning hair, dry skin, bloating, low- libido, poor focus, cold hands and feet,[26] micronutrient deficiencies,[32] and clinical or subclinical hypothyroidism/underactive thyroid. It is important for women to note that hypothyroidism can be brought on by a major life and hormonal change, such as pregnancy and postpartum, or perimenopause and menopause.

The key in healing Hashimoto's and in overcoming its younger cousin, hypothyroidism, lies in early detection.

Recommended labs to detect Hashimoto's Disease and thyroid issues of all types include:

- TSH
- Free T3
- Free T4
- Thyroid peroxidase (TPO) antibodies
- Thyroglobulin (TG) antibodies
- Reverse T3

Once your doctor has a better picture of your thyroid health, specific nutritional and lifestyle recommendations based on those findings can be made. Many integrative functional medicine doctors will recommend an elimination diet to discover food sensitivities and usually take the patient off all inflammatory foods, especially gluten. Supplements and lifestyle changes may also be recommended.

2. Leaky Gut

As discussed in Chapter 6: ENRICH, leaky gut often goes undiagnosed because of two main reasons:

- Many of its early symptoms are so common, such as bloating, indigestion, and constipation, that many people consider those symptoms to be "normal."
- Your diagnostician must know how to connect the symptoms' dots and order the correct labs to diagnose it correctly.

Recommended labs to detect leaky gut include:

- Celiac panel
- Complete stool analysis
- Lipopolysaccharide (LPS) test
- Zonulin test
- IgG food sensitivity test
- Urine organic acid test

By learning its early symptoms, causal factors, and preventative techniques, you can help protect yourself. See Chapter 6 for more information.

3. Metabolic Disease Including Pre-Diabetes and Blood Sugar Issues

Many patients have metabolic ailments, including insulin

resistance/pre-diabetes and blood sugar issues that have been sapping their energy for years.

Metabolic ailments like these typically have their roots in chronic stress, leaky gut, and an overly processed and/or an imbalanced diet. Genetics may also play a role.[33]

Recommended labs to detect these issues include:

- Fasting blood glucose
- Fasting insulin
- Hemoglobin A1C
- Fructosamine
- Advanced cholesterol panel
- HOMA
- C-peptide
- Leptin
- Adiponectin
- hsCRP

If we catch it early enough, these issues can be remedied with specific diet and lifestyle changes, such as removing sugar and most starches, eating whole, unprocessed foods, practicing meal frequency, specific supplementation, implementation of a regular exercise program, and reducing stress. Again, once your doctor has your lab results, customized recommendations can be made.

4. Candida Overgrowth

Candida overgrowth takes place when the natural fungus known as Candida albicans overtakes the good bacteria in your gut.[34] This can happen when your good gut bacteria are compromised through poor diet, antibiotic use, stress, etc., and leads to a host of unpleasant symptoms including bloating, gas, yeast infections, thrush, severe sugar and starch cravings, and other fungal infections.

Candida is common in women (especially those with recurring yeast infections and/or with leaky gut) and is often easy to resolve using diet and specific herbal and nutritional therapies.

Recommended labs to detect Candida overgrowth include:

- Candida IgG, IgA, IgM antibodies
- Complete blood count
- Complete stool analysis
- Urine organic acid test
- Heavy metals test (this may be ordered as heavy metals and Candida overgrowth often exist simultaneously)

The typical functional medicine approach to Candida is to starve the overgrowth by taking away sugars and starches (its main forms of fuel), rebuilding gut health and bacterial balance, and possibly use of supplements or herbal medicine that support normal fungal balance. Every doctor will have their own recommendations based on your unique symptoms, history, and lab results.

5. Inflammation

If you have found yourself unable to overcome specific symptoms, such as skin conditions, depression, digestive issues, headaches, insomnia, blood sugar issues, etc., you can bet there is some sort of infection, stress, or toxin creating a chronic inflammatory state. As discussed in Step 5: Enrich, chronic inflammation is at the root of nearly all chronic diseases, from diabetes and heart disease to psoriasis and cancer, and often stems from a gut-health issue. The trick is being able to isolate the cause of that inflammation, so the correct treatment program can be implemented.

Recommended labs to detect inflammation:

- ANA
- Complete stool analysis
- Ferritin
- hsCRP
- Homocysteine

6. Hormonal Imbalance

This is a big one for women of all ages, but especially those in their thirties, forties, and beyond. Your hormonal health can suffer for a variety of reasons, including lack of sleep, natural shifts (such as postpartum or perimenopause), stress, environmental toxins (such as endocrine-disrupting chemicals), dietary issues, gut health, and toxic load to name a few. Though it can be a complicated topic, one thing is for sure; if your hormones are out of whack, you're going to feel it in your physical, mental, emotional, and spiritual body. The first step to getting your hormones under control is to get a clear picture of your current hormonal makeup.

From a functional medicine perspective, this means more than just a simple blood or salivary test. Instead, or in addition to, we use advanced urinary panels to test your entire range of hormones, including levels of beneficial or non-beneficial estrogen plus how your body is methylating hormones, the health of your adrenals, and testing for any DNA oxidative damage. Once we have that full picture, we can recommend the best course of action to get your hormonal health back on track.

Recommended labs to detect hormonal imbalances:

- Dried urine test for comprehensive hormones (DUTCH test)
- FSH
- LH
- Testosterone

- Free testosterone
- Sex hormone binding globulin
- Estradiol
- Estriol
- Progesterone

7. Autoimmune Disease

Autoimmune diseases, conditions in which the body attacks its own healthy tissues, have become a growing epidemic in the last fifty years. These conditions are the result of chronic inflammation, typically rooted in gut-health issues that lead to compromised immunity, and are all too common in women young and old. Autoimmune diseases I see often in practice include psoriasis, lupus, ulcerative colitis, Crohn's Disease, Hashimoto's Disease (listed above), rheumatoid arthritis, celiac disease, scleroderma, Sjogren's syndrome, and multiple sclerosis (among others). The unfortunate thing is these conditions often go undiagnosed for years until they are at an advanced stage. The good news is you can often treat autoimmune conditions without completely relying on medication if you and your doctor know what symptoms to look for, what lab work to order to identify imbalances, and how to use integrative functional medicine to bring the body back to a balanced state of health. Despite what modern medicine would have us believe, I have seen even advanced cases of autoimmune disease go into remission using this approach, so it is never too late to start pruning.

Recommended labs if you are dealing with autoimmune disease:

- ANA
- Autoimmune panel
- Celiac panel
- Complete stool analysis
- Lipopolysaccharide (LPS) test
- Zonulin test
- IgG food sensitivity test
- Urine organic acid test
- Fasting blood glucose
- Fasting insulin
- Hemoglobin A1C
- Vitamin D
- MTHFR genes
- Homocysteine
- B12
- CBC
- CMP
- Ferritin
- Iron saturation
- Epstein Barr virus titers
- Herpes simplex titers

- Dried urine test for comprehensive hormones (DUTCH test)
- Genomic testing
- Micronutrient testing
- Heavy Metal testing
- Mycotoxin testing

Other Common Underdiagnosed Conditions for Women to Be Aware Of:

- Heavy metal toxicity—as discussed in Step 4: Weed, heavy metals are insidious and can be found in our water, cleaning products, kitchen supplies, personal care products, environment, food such as fish and seafood, and even dental materials (yes, those silver fillings that release mercury vapor every time you chew are, indeed, bad news[35]). Symptoms of exposure can vary from low energy and skin conditions to mood swings and poor gut health.
- Lyme disease and related co-infections—an epidemic in the Northeast and upper Midwest that can affect anyone, anywhere, this disease often goes undetected or misdiagnosed for years due to its complex and ever-changing symptoms. Advanced lab work is crucial in rooting out this vicious, shape-shifting disease.
- Mycotoxin exposure—mycotoxins come from molds and fungi often found growing indoors, such as in homes or office buildings. Though severe symptoms, such as asthma and hives, are hard to ignore, more subtle symptoms can

include lowered immunity, poor digestive health, hypersensitivity, headaches, chronic fatigue, and chronic colds or flu (to name but a few).

- Epstein Barr virus (EBV)—is an easily transmittable disease often misdiagnosed as a variety of fatigue-like ailments. It is a controversial disease in terms of diagnostics and treatment options, but a very real one that can be detected with the right lab tests and resolved.

- Small intestinal bacterial overgrowth (SIBO)—this is different from leaky gut in that it stems from an overgrowth of "bad" bacteria in the small intestine. Symptoms include diarrhea, loose stool, nausea, bloating, joint pain, weight loss, fatigue, and rashes. Only the correct lab work will tell you and your doctor whether it's SIBO or another digestive issue.

ADVANCED LAB PANEL CHECKLIST

For efficiency and convenience, I have provided a comprehensive list of the advanced lab tests commonly used in functional medicine below to detect nutrient deficiencies and other diseases. A downloadable version is also available in the resources section.

- Advanced lipid panel
- ANA
- Autoimmune panel
- B12

- Candida IgG, IgM, and IgA antibodies
- CBC
- Celiac panel
- CMP
- Complete stool analysis
- DUTCH test
- Epstein Barr virus antibodies
- Fasting blood glucose
- Fasting insulin
- Ferritin
- Food Sensitivity IgG Testing
- Free T3
- Free T4
- Genomic testing
- GGT
- Heavy metals test
- Hemoglobin A1C
- Herpes simplex test
- Homocysteine
- hsCRP
- Iron saturation
- LPS test
- Lyme and co-infection testing
- Micronutrient testing
- Mycotoxin testing
- Organic acid testing
- Pharmacogenetic testing

- Reverse T3
- SIBO breath test
- TG antibodies
- TPO antibodies
- TSH
- Zonulin test

HOW TO ASSEMBLE YOUR ULTIMATE HEALTHCARE PROVIDER TEAM

First and foremost, I recommend you seek out an experienced functional medicine physician who can help you navigate your health challenges from an integrative perspective.

Though there are many types of experienced and qualified integrative practitioners out there, integrative functional medicine physicians know how to work with medications and other medical issues within the framework of detoxification, supplementation, and pathology, and have the licensing to order the correct lab tests you need to prune those underlying causal factors.

However, a medical doctor, even a progressive one, should not be the only provider on your team. Other integrative providers to consider may include:

- An acupuncturist or doctor of Oriental medicine—acupuncture is extremely effective for hormonal balancing, pain management, fertility, immunity, and has been proven effective for a host of other health concerns.

- A chiropractor—chiropractors specialize in fixing subluxations of the spine and helping patients maintain overall health. Chiropractic treatment can help with a wide range ailments from back and neck pain to digestive disorders and even anxiety.

- A nutritionist or holistic dietitian to help you design a custom eating plan.

- A naturopath for in-depth detoxification strategies and other nature-based healing solutions.

- A Muscle Activation Technique (MAT™) practitioner—Muscle Activation Technique is a non-invasive form of targeted exercise that assists in correcting muscular imbalances, joint instability, and range-of-motion issues in people of all ages. It is practiced by physical therapists, chiropractors, massage therapists, and other healthcare practitioners.

- A massage therapist for stress relief, pain, and lymphatic drainage.

- A health coach—many functional medicine physicians have health coaches on staff to help keep patients on track and assist with education.

- A homeopath—for specific areas of detoxification and emotional healing.

- A holistic psychologist, counselor, or therapist for emotional healing.

Some integrative clinics have a variety of practitioners to serve you under one roof, others will refer you to trusted providers, or you may have to seek out your own team of experts.

HOW TO FIND A FUNCTIONAL MEDICINE PHYSICIAN

Though the term "functional medicine" is creating a lot of buzz, not all self-proclaimed "functional medicine physicians" have the same level of training and expertise.

To begin your search, visit the Institute of Functional Medicine website: www.ifm.org to find certified providers in your area. The functional medicine certification is an important qualifier as it will help ensure you are working with a doctor who has an in-depth understanding of integrative and functional medicine and how to get to the root cause of your ailments.

Next, visit their websites and find out what areas of health they specialize in and to get an overall feel for the practice. If it looks like the doctor may be a fit, call the patient coordinator and ask about the doctor's approach to healing and whether they have experience and success treating your condition and symptoms. You already know a lot about your health from reading this book, and you can use that knowledge to ask a few basic questions about their approach and discover if the doctor and staff seem open-minded and progressive, and if the practice aligns with your health values and goals.

Some questions to ask the patient coordinator may include:

- How long has the doctor been practicing functional medicine?
- What types of conditions does she or he treat?
- Does the doctor specialize in a particular condition?
- Can you tell me a little about the doctor's approach to diet and nutrition?
- How will we communicate if I become a patient?
- What types of diagnostic tests are used in determining causal factors?
- What will be expected of me as a patient if I partner with your clinic?

If you like what you hear on the phone, then take the next step and schedule your initial appointment.

Keep in mind, because they work within a different model, some providers may be out-of-network, and not all providers accept insurance. Some may offer a membership-based practice, where you pay a fee every month that covers all your care; some may have program fees; some may have some services covered by insurance; while others may charge by the hour for a visit.

Though these pricing structures may differ from what you are used to, I would encourage you not to be deterred. Insurance companies make it incredibly difficult (if not impossible) for doctors to spend the amount of time needed with a patient to get to the root cause of their ailments. Hence, this is why so many doctors are bound to the seven-minute visit and haste with the prescription pad.

Think of this as an investment in you. Ultimately, you will wind up saving time, money, and heartache in the long term, because you won't be feeling sick all the time. That—your health, your peace of mind, and your sense of value—is worth everything.

The labs I recommend in this chapter can be done with a conventional doctor, but I highly recommend you seek out a functional medicine physician for three reasons:

1. They will know how to identify your symptoms correctly and order the right tests (which will save you time and money).

2. They know how to interpret the labs even if your results are "within normal range."

3. They know how to use an integrative functional medicine approach to get to the root cause of imbalances.

Just like in a garden, pruning and encouraging the process of ongoing health is a process.

If, after implementing the steps in this book and giving them some time to work, you continue to feel unwell or just not yourself, come back to this chapter for help seeking out a functional medicine physician. A good doctor, aka "professional pruner," will help you trim back the overgrowth, reignite that spark of energy you have been missing, and accelerate your journey to full Bloom.

With the pruning process complete (or underway), we move onto the final step in the Bloom process, Step 7: BALANCE. Here, you will learn the guiding principles and best practices you can implement to stay the course of health as the seasons of your life unfold. See you there!

Pruning Action Items (grab those shears!):

- Go through the symptoms of nutrients deficiencies and clinical/subclinical conditions discussed in this chapter, and see if any apply to your current experience.
- If so, use the tips provided and seek out a certified functional medicine physician.
- Talk to your doctor about having labs done, as outlined in

this chapter, to check for the deficiencies and conditions discussed.

- Continue to update your lab results at least twice a year (or per doctor's recommendations) to establish a baseline.

PRUNE Resources at nourishmedicine.com/bloomresources:

- Access The Institute of Functional Medicine's "Find a Practitioner" tool
- The Vitamin D Council's Sun Exposure Recommendations By Skin Type
- Advanced Functional Medicine Lab Checklist Download

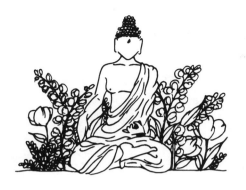

CHAPTER 8

Step 7: BALANCE— Easy Hacks to Stay the Course

———

One of the features of a well-balanced garden is resiliency. If one year is plagued by heavy rains and the next brings drought, the tended garden will survive and continue to produce. Likewise, the six steps we have been applying to your Bloom process will help sustain you through life's hardships, slip-ups, and times of imbalance. *We will all face hardships, slip-ups, and times of imbalance.* This is when you will tap into those established reservoirs of self-care, nutrition, attitude cultivation, gut health, and stress management to sustain you through life's storms. Emotionally trying times also call for an increase in flexibility, mindfulness, and care of your spiritual body.

Step 7: BALANCE will introduce my favorite hacks you can use to maintain your newfound physical, emotional, and spiritual strength in the face of trying life circumstances.

TIFFANY'S STORY

Tiffany, a stressed-out single mom with a high-pressure job, came to me with many of the health issues I see frequently in my practice. She was feeling fatigued, bloated, and experienced frequent bouts of stress-induced illness. When we ran her lab tests, we discovered she was deficient in a several vitamins and nutrients, she had dysbiosis (a type of inflammatory gut infection) and was suffering from a slew of food sensitivities.

We discussed options, and I put her on the program outlined in this book. After just a few months, she saw marked improvements; then, she hit a rough patch when things at work went downhill, and her stress levels went through the roof. Before we worked together, this type of stressful situation would have landed Tiffany back in bed with extreme fatigue and digestive stress. However, that's not what happened this time.

When I followed up with her, not only had her blood markers improved, but she was also pleased to report she hadn't been sick at all. She had gained an amazing amount of resiliency by working to heal her gut—and by extension, her immune system. She had also taken deliberate steps to establish a self-care regime and support system, which all gave her a greater ability to weather life's storms *and* remain strong.

If, like Tiffany, the guiding principles of your life prioritize growth and caring for yourself and your body, it's going to be easier for you to recover from less-than-optimal circumstances.

THE DANCE OF REAL LIFE

The capacity to be flexible and resilient is one of the best gifts we can give ourselves. Life is going to happen, we are going to have work challenges, family crises, relationship woes, ups and downs, and unexpected change in our lives. In each of these moments, we have a choice to either be hard and rigid *or* gentle and flexible with ourselves.

What happens when we live in a rigid state of perfectionism?

It makes us brittle to the point where a slight setback is enough to break us. In a state of expansiveness, we are flexible enough to see setbacks as opportunities for transformation. They offer us a chance to reflect on what is, what may need to change, and what matters.

A flexible, expansive attitude can be especially helpful in weathering a health crisis. For example, I often challenge my patients to view their symptoms as a blessing instead of a curse, because a symptom is your body's way of telling you something is not right and needs to be fixed. So, even seemingly unpleasant experiences can be incredible opportunities for change and transformation, and we are willing to see them in that light.

It's similar to dancing. When you dance with a partner, you follow each other moving together in a coordinated and flexible way always staying in equilibrium. There is give and take in such a way that both dancers can express themselves. It's important to be able to bring yourself back to your center, but almost equally important is the ability to be flexible and strong in the face of life's challenges.

MINDFULNESS

Mindfulness is the state of being conscious or aware of something in the present moment without judgment.

Though mindfulness has gained a lot of cultural currency lately, it is not a new practice. In fact, our grandparents and ancestors practiced mindfulness every day by focusing their attention on one thing at a time.

However, the pace of life has quickened, and endless distractions from devices, media, and other sources have taken us from the present moment and into a chronic state of unfocused chaos. This state of constant distraction and multitasking feeds into that fight-or-flight stress response discussed in previous chapters, and has been proven to damage our brains by shrinking gray matter, reducing IQ, and impairing our ability to focus and perform effectively.[1]

Thus, the surging popularity of mindfulness helps counterbalance those effects. Research has also shown that mindfulness practices, and specifically meditation, can help:[2,3]

- Reduce pain
- Quell anxiety and depression
- Improve sleep quality
- Improve blood sugar

Though I encourage patients to explore meditation (see resources section for more information), anyone can practice mindfulness in any area of their life any time by following one or more of these three simple principles:

1. Take an inventory of your senses: What are you seeing, smelling, tasting, touching, and hearing?

2. You can also remain focused on your breathing by counting seconds during which you breathe in and out. This is especially useful when walking or meditating.

3. Finding a mantra can be useful, too, especially in tense situations or when you feel fearful. It could be as simple as the word "peace" or more specific like "I have abundance in my life."

The basic idea is to be curious and focused on the present moment, and if you find your thoughts drifting away, gently bring your attention back to what you're doing. It's that easy and will help you let go of the worry and stress from living in the past or future.

Start by practicing mindfulness for three minutes a day and work up from there. See resources section for helpful apps.

MINDFUL EATING—AN EXAMPLE OF EVERYDAY MINDFULNESS IN ACTION

How does one eat mindfully? By engaging as many senses as possible in the eating process. Remember to chew for at least twenty seconds!

- Look at your food. What are the colors like? What kinds of shapes do you see?

- Smell the aroma. Is the food hot or cold?

- Taste it. What is the texture like? Is it sweet, bitter, or savory?

ENERGY MEDICINE PRACTICES—CARING
FOR YOUR ENERGETIC BODY

In addition to the various other techniques for enhanced spiritual well-being outlined in this book, energy medicine practices can make a world of difference in helping us maintain balance.

Though energy medicine is often considered "esoteric" in the West, these ancient practices have been revered for centuries in Eastern systems of medicine, such as traditional Chinese medicine, and Ayurvedic medicine—the traditional medicine of India.

In a nutshell, energy medicine looks at the flow of electricity, or "energy," running through your body as a reflection of overall health. If this sounds out there, keep in mind that the human body is as much (if not more) electrical in nature as it is biological. Think about how we track heart rate variability using electrocardiograms (EKGs), or how we observe brain waves through electroencephalogram (EEGs), or the electrical nature of the nervous system. However you choose to look at it, it is clear human beings are fundamentally governed by energy, and it is important to keep that energy in good alignment.

The following are some time-tested and scientifically proven methods for rebalancing your stress response and maintaining a resilient energetic body.

Yoga: Most people are familiar with yoga—the mind-body practice that originated in India, in which you move and stretch, practice breath work, and focus your mind. It was originally invented to loosen up the body so practitioners could sit for hours in meditation, but it's also a darn good workout. There are many different forms of yoga—from static, strength-based endurance stretches to flow sequences to meditation-based practices—so I encourage you to try out a few at local studios or online, to see which style you enjoy

Health-wise, yoga has been shown to:

- Positively impact the stress response[4]
- And has been linked to easing depression and anxiety[5]

Qigong: Qigong is an ancient Chinese practice that uses coordinated body posture and movement, along with breath work, meditation, and martial arts training using slow, flowing movement.

Health-wise, it has been shown to:

- Decrease hypertension[6]
- Decrease pain[7]
- And help lower stress[8]

Qigong has many forms, the most well-known in the United States being tai chi. Its slow pace and focused movement make it an excellent choice for those seeking to relax and focus the mind while they move.

Qoya: Qoya is a new expressive movement practice rooted in dance and yoga. The foundational belief is that it helps a woman remember she is wise, wild, and free. It is an empowering and therapeutic movement practice that allows participants to express the truth of their bodies, while accessing the wisdom of yoga and other spiritual practices. Classes are only for women, and the focus is on freedom and reveling in your body. Highly recommended!

Acupuncture: Acupuncture is a centuries-old traditional Chinese medicine system that looks at the body as a collection of meridians and energy pathways. There are thousands of studies about the efficacy of acupuncture (see resources); it's basically good for everything including relieving stress. The needles used are hair-thin and, when inserted, feel like a gentle tap on the skin. It is not painful, rather deeply relaxing. One of my patients who has a very demanding job, swears by her weekly acupuncture session as a key to creating resiliency in her life.

Reiki: Reiki is a Japanese modality of healing touch or "laying on of hands" as a way to balance energies in the body. The reiki practitioner will hover their hands above specific energy points and blockages in the body to facilitate rebalancing.

While it may sound a little touchy-feely, it has been shown to have objective results:

- Reiki helps to decrease stress and anxiety, and promote better mood[9]
- Decreases pain allowing for greater relaxation[10]

You can find a reiki practitioner through professional organizations like the International Association of Reiki Professionals (see resources for more information).

Craniosacral Therapy: Craniosacral therapy is another form of bodywork that uses therapeutic touch to gently adjust the cranium and the synarthrodial joint to manipulate the flow of cerebrospinal fluid. It helps to release tension and can offer a relaxing and healing experience. Patients swear by it for a number ailments, including headaches, jaw pain, and even colicky babies. Many doctors, chiropractors, and other practitioners offer cranial work, or you can find a specialist through various associations (see resources).

Massage: Records of massage as a healing art go back three thousand years, and range from China to Persia to Egypt.

There are many different types and forms of massage to address a variety of ailments, from muscle tension and TMG to lymphatic drainage stimulation. I recommend getting a massage once a month (or more frequently if you can swing it) to bring you back into balance, and help support your personal restoration and replenishment.

Being in Nature: While we talked about the benefits of being in nature and "earthing" in earlier chapters, it bears repeating as earthing is a form of energetic medicine. Being in contact with the earth, looking at nature, and even imagining nature can help reset your stress response and refill your reservoir. It's important to be deliberate about spending time in nature every day—even a ten-minute evening walk or time spent playing in the dirt with your children will make a world of difference.

QUICK WAYS TO FIND BALANCE DURING A STRESSFUL DAY OR MOMENT

Even when it feels like stress is taking over, there is always something you can do to bring yourself back into a balanced, restorative state. Some ideas include:

- Take a short walk outside.

- Practice deep belly breathing. Breathing deeply in through the nose to your belly while now allowing your shoulders to rise, then exhaling fully through your mouth. Repeat ten to twenty times.

- Use your HeartMath app to help guide you back to restorative mode.

- Watch a funny video and laugh your heart out.

- Give yourself a little extra support by calling a friend or family member for quick chat.

- Have a five-minute dance party to your favorite, uplifting tune.

- Write down some gratitudes.

- Go outside and walk around barefoot. Even just a few minutes of earthing can help you feel more grounded.

- Repeat your chosen mantra. For example, "I have abundance in my life." or "All is well within."

WHICH BALANCING HACKS WILL WORK BEST FOR YOU?

Use your intuition to choose what kinds of energy practices are best for you. What sparks your interest? What calls to your spirit? Be adventurous and try something new!

Write down one or two energy medicine practices you would like to try, then get out there and give them your best shot.

Congratulations! By completing this final step to maintaining the resilient health you have created throughout the seven-step process, you are finally ready to Bloom. Before we move into our last chapter together, I invite you to go back to the beginning of our journey: page 1, "The Mindful Gardener," and re-read this piece with fresh eyes. This short exercise will help you get the most out of our last chapter as we come together one last time to solidify all you have learned and celebrate your new spark for life.

Balancing Action Items:

- Cultivate that attitude of expansion, and keep your reminders handy for when bad-days strike.
- Start incorporating mindfulness into your everyday experiences.
- Seek out the healing energy practice or practices that work best for you, and engage in them regularly.

BALANCE Resources at nourishmedicine.com/bloomresources:

- "How Acupuncture Works, an Article on the Efficacy of Acupuncture" by The University of California, San Diego
- "Find a Practitioner" resources and links
- Find a Balancing Practice resources and links

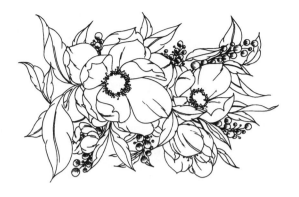

CHAPTER 9

BLOOM—
Empowerment,
Grace, and Joy

—

A beautiful patient of mine, Maya, first came to see me when she was about thirty-seven. She had a demanding career, a marriage on the rocks, and a whole host of physical symptoms. She suffered from thyroid disease, pre-diabetes, food sensitivities, several nutrient deficiencies, and gut dysfunction. She was also a complete workaholic—always on, always sacrificing herself for her work, and always giving to others. When she wasn't at work, she was pouring herself into saving her marriage to little avail.

When Maya first came to me, we talked about what she wanted to create for herself and her life. She told me she wanted happiness, joy, and freedom, so those were the seeds we sowed as steps or guiding principles. From there, we worked to restore her gut, and we thoroughly pruned the physical and emotional overgrowth preventing her from reaching full Bloom.

Within a short period, she had built up her health and strength enough to leave her toxic marriage and begin a new life of happiness, joy, and freedom. She found her balance, and she is now able to check her inner compass and figure out when she is losing her true path, so she can return to equilibrium.

Note I said, "return to equilibrium." Maya still struggles to maintain her balance. We all do, and that's my point: Achieving optimal wellness and coming into full Bloom is a journey—not a fixed destination. We will always be growing and working through new phases within this cycle as we gain more skills to continue fostering lifelong health.

Maya and I still work together regularly, checking her labs, tweaking her diet, and figuring out ways for her to better manage the stressors in her life. This demonstrates the value in developing a good relationship with a functional medicine physician, so they can check your labs every three to six months and help eliminate any imbalances.

Beyond that, it is crucial you continue to fill your reservoir with daily stress management practices and spiritual work, while making self-care, hobbies, and friendships a priority.

THE JOURNEY IS THE DESTINATION

Health, just like anything we seek to create in life, will always be a process. Gardens move through different seasons of planting, growing, harvesting, and resting. Likewise, in life, there are times of growth—when we are rapidly putting forth leaves and blossoms—and there are times when we need to slow down and take in extra nourishment. We may need to amend our gut soil, prune emotional overgrowth, or spend some time pulling out those toxic weeds—which will always pop up. The process, just like our own personal growth, is never-ending, and that's just as it should be.

Now that you understand what you need to do for yourself, for your personal garden, it's not as overwhelming, is it? When you keep your intentions and goals in the forefront, have a system in place, and understand your landscape, you can simply apply these steps as guiding principles and continue with life. That's how you foster your seeds throughout the seasons and ensure your own prosperity and well-being for life.

Remember, too, you can work smarter, not harder. Picking up a hobby is a great way to do this. Join a choir, take art classes, cook for yourself or your family—seek out connection, fulfillment, and health in your activities. You can multitask (in a healthy way) on your path to well-being.

Stay with your why. It is crucial you not lose sight of what you want to create in your life. Remember the plan you made for your garden, and remember that, while you may need to replenish the soil in one area, it may be time to sow seeds in another.

THERE IS NO "PERFECT HEALTH" IN THIS PROCESS

At the risk of sounding like a broken record, I want to remind you there is no "perfection" in this Bloom process—but there is also no failure. It is just a process, and once you are empowered within this process, and you know what steps to take, you can just adjust as necessary, so you can truly care for yourself.

As we discussed at the beginning of the book, when your plants aren't growing well you don't freak out and blame the plants; you figure out *why* they are not growing and take steps to fix the problem. You can be happy, healthy, and fulfilled, even while you're still working on "unfinished" areas in your health and life. Life is an ongoing process, and that is as it should be.

ADJUSTING COURSE ALONG THE WAY

Let's look at a few different scenarios bound to come up in a yearly cycle, and how you can use the steps outlined in each phase of the Bloom process to deal with them effectively and stay the course.

Scenario 1: The Holidays Throw You Off Track

When this happens, it's time to revisit the Nourish, Enrich, and Prune principles.

- If you've put on some weight and/or feel bloated, consider regaining your nutritional equilibrium by doing an elimination diet for two weeks, and give some extra care to your gut.
- If your immunity is low, look at what you may need to prune.
- If you're exhausted and low on energy, pay careful attention to your sleep cycle and self-care regime.

Scenario 2: Work or Family Life Gets Crazy and Wears You Down

In this more-than-likely scenario, shift your focus to Enriching your gut, your Root system, and your Balance.

- The minute you feel "used up," you know it's time to refill your cup. Go back to the energetic medicine practices discussed in Chapter 8 and schedule some time to partake in a reiki session, acupuncture treatment, yoga class, etc.

- This should also signal the need to lean on your established support system for extra help around the house, with the kids, etc.
- Be mindful of your gut health, as the added stress can take a toll on your digestion and immunity.

Scenario 3: Travel Is Making It Difficult to Nourish Yourself Properly

When business or pleasure trips call, it's time to tap your reservoirs and prepare to Weed when you return home.

- During these times, it is important to RELAX and remember food is important, BUT it's not everything. If you have taken the steps to fill your reservoir, your body will be healthy and resilient despite a few days of less-than-optimal eating. Rather, focus your attention on your stress levels and emotional well-being. Be sure you're taking time for those self-care practices, even if it means bringing your gratitude journal with you and/or using an app to meditate in your hotel room before bed.
- Supplements, like probiotics and even organic, powdered green drinks, can be extremely helpful on the road to keep your immunity and nutrient levels up.
- Travel can also cause extra exposure to electromagnetic

frequencies (EMFs) from air travel, airport scanners (you can opt for a pat down, by the way), etc. So be sure to find a park or patch of grass where you can practice a little earthing and discharge some of that excess electricity.

DR. ALEX'S MUST-HAVE SUPPLEMENTS FOR TRAVEL:

- Activated charcoal—this natural product is used by doctors and hospitals for food poisoning and works wonders to absorb any toxins or impurities in the gut.[1]

- Probiotics to maintain immunity and gut health on the road.[2]

- Digestive enzymes to help you get the most out of restaurant food.

- Melatonin—a natural way to curb jet lag and help you get more sleep away from home.[3]

- Organic green drink powders for a convenient shot of phytonutrients anywhere.

- Echinacea—research has proven taking echinacea while traveling can help reduce your chances of "airplane colds" and other travel-related respiratory illnesses.[4]

Bottom line: If you are aware of your needs and the way your body works, you can care for it better no matter what your circumstances.

ESSENTIAL SUPPLEMENTS FOR THE FULL BLOOM LIFESTYLE:

I recommend these essential supplements to all my patients to help maintain health and longevity. In the interest of purity, safety, and efficacy I recommend purchasing professional-grade supplement brands from your functional medicine physician.

- A quality multivitamin to ensure you receive adequate nutrients, even on those "off" days.

- Fish oil supplement to boost your intake of omega-3 fatty acids, support healthy skin, cognitive function, heart health, and keep inflammation in check.[5] Look for an EPA (eicosapentaenoic acid) and DHA (docosahexaenoic acid) combination of 1000 mg.

- Multi-strain probiotic to maintain a diversified and healthy gut microbiome and promote healthy immune function. Look for a multi-strain formula with around 50 million CFUs, prebiotics, and no added sugars, artificial sweeteners, fillers, or preservatives.

- Magnesium glycinate to promote bone health, sleep, heart health, digestion and elimination, blood sugar levels, muscle health, prevent headaches, and much more. Be sure to choose the glycinate form of magnesium for its superior absorbability and digestive health benefits.[6] I typically recommend 300 mg daily taken before bed.

- Vitamin D3 with K2 to promote bone health, immunity, hormonal balance, and mental and emotional well-being.[7,8] I typically recommend 5000 ius daily, but check with your doctor based on your current levels and lifestyle.

- A protein powder—benefits of a daily protein shake or smoothie include balanced blood sugar, easier weight management, and a nice nutrient boost. My favorite protein powders include organic pea protein isolate, organic hemp protein, hydrolyzed grass-fed beef protein powder, and hydrolyzed grass-fed collagen.

Human beings are social creatures. Because of that, we gain a lot of joy and satisfaction from helping others. As you continue through this process of Blooming, you also set yourself to go out into the world and serve from a place of genuineness. When you are taking care of yourself, it creates a ripple effect; your care for yourself spills over as a greater ability to care for others.

My grandmother, for example, lived to be 103 and spent every single day of her life volunteering in her community. She was service-oriented, true, but she cared for herself and lived in a way that allowed her to remain healthy. Her service to community also built her up by giving her connection and purpose. She could not have given so much to so many had she not first cared for herself.

When we give back to others from a place of strength, it creates a positive feedback loop that nourishes everyone—the bright opposite of the typical sacrificial, everything-for-everyone-else, survival-oriented lifestyle so many women feel they must live.

There are so many ways to share your harvest with the world:

- For some people, that's working in community gardens.

- For others, it's volunteering at a food pantry.
- For many, doing charity work is fulfilling.
- Some enjoy tutoring or volunteering at the YMCA.
- Others make a point to help their neighbors with everyday chores.
- If, for you, it means just being present in your life, and sharing it moment by moment with the ones you love, that's excellent, too.

While volunteer work is easily measurable, there are as many ways to share your gifts as there are people in this world. You can give your time, your talent, your resources, or some combination of all three—but by caring for yourself, you will be able to do it bigger and better.

Instead of being forced to give until you can give no more, when you care for yourself you create a more reciprocal arrangement. You are always refilling your cup, and therefore, you always have more to share with your family members, your children, and your community. When we embrace that truth, our service comes from an authentic place of generosity, instead of a place of martyrdom.

A dedication to self-care also allows us to empower other people (especially other women) on their journey: "If she can do it, I can too." We need to spread that around like confetti!

You should be the receiver of good things. Only once you have accepted that you *deserve* care can you move into a position of helping others. When you accept you *deserve* to have the things you want in your life—health, joy, freedom, creativity, and all those other seeds we choose to plant—you can create goodness, beauty, inspiration, empowerment, and happiness in everything and everyone you touch.

YOU ARE THE MASTER OF YOUR GENETICS

Lifestyle is hugely epigenetic—meaning, we have the power to control how our genes are expressed. In other words, your genes aren't your destiny, your environment is. The way that you choose to live your life, the way that you choose to engage with your thoughts, your beliefs, and all the practices we've talked about, are epigenetic modifiers. Ultimately, YOU are in serious control of your destiny.

FULL BLOOM

As this phase in our journey together ends, remember every part of this process can be repeated as needed:

- You can Sow new seeds as your previous seeds come to Bloom.
- You can Weed out just about any toxin that comes up.
- You can Prune, with the help of your integrative healthcare team, whenever you need to.
- You can always spread your Root system deeper and wider.

- And there is always time and reason to Balance, Enrich, and Nourish yourself further.

But always remember your why. *Why* are you doing this? Ultimately, you want to have a flourishing garden, full of whatever seeds you choose to plant. To achieve that, however, you will need to keep your focus and stay strong—and returning to this book as needed is a terrific way to do that.

Remember the story of the Hurried Gardener and the Mindful Gardener I asked you to re-read with fresh eyes? The moral is: You can't plant seeds in a garden, walk away, and expect it to grow. You must make a commitment to care for it, observe it, and tend to it regularly. It's a constant process of amending, nourishing, weeding, planting, pruning, and enriching—but just look at the beautiful results!

"When autumn came, the mindful gardener carefully gathered all the seeds from her remaining plants to use the following year, and had more than enough seed left to share the precious gifts of her little garden with her friend and the greater world."

THREE BLOSSOMS ON THE BRANCH

- Remember your Why, always.

- Every step can be repeated as often as necessary.

- There is no perfection; it's a constant search for balance and beauty.

BLOOM Resources at nourishmedicine.com/bloomresources:

- Download the Essential Supplements for the Full Bloom Lifestyle Supplement Guide
- Access the Life in Bloom Facebook community for ongoing support

Acknowledgements

Writing a book is no small endeavor. This book is truly a lifetime in the making, and it couldn't have been born without the help, support, inspiration, and love from so many.

My profound thanks and gratitude to:

Danny, for being my anchor—since the day we met, you have supported all of my ideas and dreams, and you jumped in wholeheartedly to co-create a life that reflected our vision and values.

Camila and Lucho, for gifting me with the indescribable, heart-filling love of motherhood, and for filling my life with purpose, tenderness, and joy.

Mami and Papi, Ela and Lucio Varela, for always supporting my dreams and for teaching me how to navigate through life with kindness, generosity, love, and fun.

Dan and Mary Esther Carrasco, for raising an incredible son and for being so generous and supportive of our dreams as individuals and as a couple.

Diana, Mario, and Noah Carrasco, for being the extended family I always wished for.

Dora, for taking care of our family with such genuine love and care day in and day out.

James and Rachel Maskell, for encouraging me to take the leap and open my dream practice in 2012.

Kristen Boye, for being such an amazing wordsmith and for bringing my words to life with profound heart and soul.

Jenna Rainey, for your beautiful illustrations.

Dr. Mark Hyman and Dr. Andrew Weil, for planting the seeds of inspiration in my soul more than a decade ago and for bringing functional and integrative medicine to the forefront.

Dr. Christine Maren, Dr. Emily Gutierrez, Dr. Vincent Pedre, Dr. Seth Osgood, Alyse Snyder, Dr. Ben House, Dr. Iris Wingrove, Brandon O'Connor, Melissa Clough, Dr. Katriny Ikbal, and Dr. Kevin Lewis, for being amazing healers, colleagues, and friends who I can always count on.

Dr. Jolene Brighten, Dr. Maya Shetreat-Klein, Dr. Mariza Snyder, Teri Cochrane, Dr. Shawn Tassone, Dr. Ann Shippy, Dr. Joe Tatta, Dr. Nicole Beurkens, Dr. Izabella Wentz, Dr. Anthony Youn, Dr. Kellyann Petrucci, Dr. V. Desaulniers, Dr. Jerry Bailey, and Dr. Pamela Langenderfer, for your friendship and for supporting my vision and encouraging me to find my voice.

JJ Virgin, for your mentorship and generosity.

Uli and Jen Iserloh, for seeing this project through with me from its infancy to its fruition.

My first mentors in medicine—Dr. David Ruiz and Dr. Robert Casanova—you taught me the art of medicine; witnessing you practice medicine the many summers I worked in your clinics during high school and college taught me *how* I wanted to be with my patients—compassionate and connected.

My beautiful "Cuban family" in Austin—Carol Wood and Jorge Garces, Ana Teresa Garces-Wood, Jorge Antonio Garces-Wood, Irene and Al Burke, Charo and Rafael Marquez, Natacha and Alexa Wagner, Tillie De Armas, Maria Teresa and David Ruiz, Chris and Robert Casanova, Ileana Casanova, Ana Pozo, Ana Hernandez, Nadya and Rafael Padilla, for teaching me we *can* create our family wherever we go; and thank you for teaching me how important food, laughter, music and dancing are for a happy, rooted, and well-lived life.

My beloved grandparents—Abuela Mercedes, Abuelo Juan, Abuelita Lilia, and Abuelito David, for filling me with so much love and so many stories. You were the first ones to teach me how important it is to listen to one another's stories.

My tíos and tías—Juan and Margaret, Tia Irma, Tio Marvin, Tia Susy, Tio Mario, Tia Ceci, Tio Junior and Tia Chela, for your love and support throughout my life.

My beautiful cousins—Juani, Vica, Stephanie, Cassie, Jackie, Michelle, Jacob, David, Mario, and Eddie, for dreaming big with me when I was a kid.

Anna María Mendéz, for your steadfast friendship since we were fourteen years old. You have always encouraged me, set me straight, and believed in me even when I haven't.

Mimi Garcia, your confidence and kick-ass attitude has inspired me to dream big and take big leaps since we met at Orchestra Camp when we were eleven.

My Rice University family—Karen, Dave, Heather, Ille, Iris, Eric, Ammar, Evan, Randy, and Tina, for encouraging me in undergrad when I set my sights on practicing integrative medicine; for believing in me back then and for encouraging me all the way until today.

The Mangos—Dr. Sonia Sosa, Dr. Suzanne Powers, Dr. Sean Zager and Dr. Karolina Dembinsky, for sharing the dream of changing the face of medicine when we were med students and for the gift of co-creating a powerfully healing HEART 2007 elective that still resonates even a decade later.

Ellie Brett, for helping me find my SPARK.

Linda Drake, for your encouragement and for connecting me to my power.

Kelly Roetto, for being the most wonderful, generous, and amazing Patient Coordinator/Wearer Of Many Hats for Nourish Medicine. You are such a blessing!

Most importantly, thank you to my incredible patients for opening your hearts and souls and for allowing me the sacred privilege of partnering with you in your journey to healing—without you, this book would not exist.

About the Author

——

ALEJANDRA CARRASCO, MD, FAAFP, FABIHM, IFM-CP, received her undergraduate degree from Rice University and earned her medical degree from the University of Texas Long School of Medicine in San Antonio. After completing a family medicine residency at Brackenridge Hospital in Austin, Texas, she went on to complete the Functional Medicine Certification Program through the Institute of Functional Medicine. In 2012 she founded Nourish Medicine, an integrative and functional medicine practice that seeks to uncover the root causes of illness and bring patients back to health and healing. Her practice website is www.nourishmedicine.com.

References

___

CHAPTER 2

1. Blackwell, Simon E., Nathaly Rius-Ottenheim, Yvonne W.M. Schulte-van Maaren, Ingrid V.E. Carlier, Victor D. Middelkoop, Frans G. Zitman, Philip Spinhoven, Emily A. Holmes, and Erik J. Giltay. "Optimism and Mental Imagery: A Possible Cognitive Marker to Promote Well-being?" Psychiatry Research. March 30, 2013. Accessed May 01, 2017. https://www.ncbi.nlm.nih.gov/pmc/articles/PMC3605581/.
2. Bardone-Cone, Anna M., Katrina Sturm, Melissa A. Lawson, D. Paul Robinson, and Roma Smith. "Perfectionism Across Stages of Recovery from Eating Disorders." The International Journal of Eating Disorders. March 2010. Accessed May 01, 2017. https://www.ncbi.nlm.nih.gov/pmc/articles/PMC2820585/.
3. Egan, S. J., T. D. Wade, and R. Shafran. "Perfectionism as a Transdiagnostic Process: A Clinical Review." Clinical Psychology Review. March 2011. Accessed May 01, 2017. http://www.ncbi.nlm.nih.gov/pubmed/20488598.
4. Friis, A. M., M. H. Johnson, R. G. Cutfield, and N. S. Consedine. "Kindness Matters: A Randomized Controlled Trial of a Mindful Self-Compassion Intervention Improves Depression, Distress, and HbA1c Among Patients With Diabetes." Diabetes Care. November 2016. Accessed May 01, 2017. https://www.ncbi.nlm.nih.gov/pubmed/27335319.

CHAPTER 3

1. Liu, Rui Hai. "Health-Promoting Components of Fruits and Vegetables in the Diet1,2." Advances in Nutrition: An International Review Journal. May 01, 2013. Accessed May 01, 2017. http://advances.nutrition.org/content/4/3/384S.full.

2. "Ivan Pavlov - Facts." Nobelprize.org. Accessed May 01, 2017. http://www.nobelprize. org/nobel_prizes/medicine/laureates/1904/pavlov-facts.html.

3. Giduck, S. A., R. M. Threatte, and M. R. Kare. "Cephalic Reflexes: Their Role in Digestion and Possible Roles in Absorption and Metabolism." The Journal of Nutrition. July 1987. Accessed May 20, 2017. https://www.ncbi.nlm.nih.gov/ pubmed/3302135.

4. Champeau, Rachel. "Changing Gut Bacteria through Diet Affects Brain Function, UCLA Study Shows." UCLA Newsroom. May 28, 2013. Accessed May 26, 2017. http://newsroom.ucla.edu/releases/changing-gut-bacteria-through-245617.

5. Watts, A. W., K. Loth, J. M. Berge, N. Larson, and D. Neumark-Sztainer. "No Time for Family Meals? Parenting Practices Associated with Adolescent Fruit and Vegetable Intake When Family Meals Are Not an Option." Journal of the Academy of Nutrition and Dietetics. May 2017. Accessed May 01, 2017. https://www.ncbi.nlm. nih.gov/pubmed/27989447.

6. MPH, Marla E. Eisenberg ScD. "Correlations Between Family Meals and Psychosocial Well-being Among Adolescents." Archives of Pediatrics & Adolescent Medicine. August 01, 2004. Accessed May 20, 2017. doi:10.1001/archpedi.158.8.792.

7. Yangabc, Yang Claire, Courtney Boenab, Karen Gerkenab, Ting Lid, and Kristen Schorppab And. "Yang Claire Yang." Proceedings of the National Academy of Sciences. January 04, 2016. Accessed May 02, 2017. doi:10.1073/pnas.1511085112.

8. Pollan, Michael. The Omnivore's Dilemma: A Natural History of Four Meals. NY, NY: Penguin Books, 2016.

9. Morell, Sally Fallon. "Broth Is Beautiful." The Weston A. Price Foundation. January 01, 2000. Accessed March 29, 2017. https://www.westonaprice.org/health-topics/ food-features/broth-is-beautiful/.

10. Fallon, Sally, Mary G. Enig, Kim Murray, and Marion Dearth. "Stocks." In Nourishing Traditions: The Cookbook That Challenges Politically Correct Nutrition and the Diet Dictocrats, 116-18. Washington, DC: NewTrends Publishing, 2005.

11. Parvez, S., K. A. Malik, S. Ah, and H. Y. Kim. "Probiotics and Their Fermented Food Products Are Beneficial for Health." Journal of Applied Microbiology. June 2006. Accessed May 01, 2017. doi:10.1111/j.1365-2672.2006.02963.x.

12. Gwirtz, Jeffrey A., and Maria Nieves Garcia-Casal. "Processing Maize Flour and Corn Meal Food Products." Annals of the New York Academy of Sciences. April 2014. Accessed May 20, 2017. doi:10.1111/nyas.12299.

13. Gupta, Raj Kishor, Shivraj Singh Gangoliya, and Nand Kumar Singh. "Reduction of Phytic Acid and Enhancement of Bioavailable Micronutrients in Food Grains." Journal of Food Science and Technology. February 2015. Accessed May 20, 2017. doi:10.1007/s13197-013-0978-y.

14. Fallon, Sally, Mary G. Enig, Kim Murray, and Marion Dearth. "Stocks." In Nourishing Traditions: The Cookbook That Challenges Politically Correct Nutrition and the Diet Dictocrats, 116-18. Washington, DC: NewTrends Publishing, 2005.

15. Pottenger, Francis M., Elaine Pottenger, and Robert T. Pottenger. Pottenger's Cats: A Study in Nutrition. La Mesa, CA (P.O. Box 2614, La Mesa 92041): Price-Pottenger Nutrition Foundation, 2009.

16. Lee, Richard B., and Irven DeVore. Man the Hunter /edited by Richard B. Lee and Irven DeVore: With the Assistance of Jill Nash-Mitchell. New Brunswick: Aldine Transaction, 1968.

17. Valenta, Rudolf, Heidrun Hochwallner, Birgit Linhart, and Sandra Pahr. "Food Allergies: The Basics." Gastroenterology. May 2015. Accessed May 20, 2017. doi:10.1053/j.gastro.2015.02.006.

18. Bischoff, Stephan C., Giovanni Barbara, Wim Buurman, Theo Ockhuizen, Jörg-Dieter Schulzke, Matteo Serino, Herbert Tilg, Alastair Watson, and Jerry M. Wells. "Intestinal Permeability – a New Target for Disease Prevention and Therapy." BMC Gastroenterology. November 18, 2014. Accessed May 20, 2017. doi:10.1186/s12876-014-0189-7.

19. David, L. A., C. F. Maurice, R. N. Carmody, D. B. Gootenberg, J. E. Button, B. E. Wolfe, A. V. Ling, A. S. Devlin, Y. Varma, M. A. Fischbach, S. B. Biddinger, R. J. Dutton, and P. J. Turnbaugh. "Diet Rapidly and Reproducibly Alters the Human Gut Microbiome." Nature. December 11, 2013. Accessed May 20, 2017. doi:10.1038/nature12820.

20. Sigthorsson, G., J. Tibble, J. Hayllar, I. Menzies, A. Macpherson, R. Moots, D. Scott, M. Gumpel, and I. Bjarnason. "Intestinal Permeability and Inflammation in Patients on NSAIDs." Gut. October 1998. Accessed May 01, 2017. https://www.ncbi.nlm.nih.gov/pmc/articles/PMC1727292/.

21. Kelly, John R., Paul J. Kennedy, John F. Cryan, Timothy G. Dinan, Gerard Clarke, and Niall P. Hyland. "Breaking down the Barriers: The Gut Microbiome, Intestinal Permeability and Stress-related Psychiatric Disorders." Frontiers in Cellular Neuroscience. October 14, 2015. Accessed May 06, 2017. doi:10.3389/fncel.2015.00392.

22. Phillips, Melissa Lee. "Gut Reaction: Environmental Effects on the Human Microbiota." Environmental Health Perspectives. May 2009. Accessed May 23, 2017. https://www.ncbi.nlm.nih.gov/pmc/articles/PMC2685866/.

23. Bischoff, Stephan C., Giovanni Barbara, Wim Buurman, Theo Ockhuizen, Jörg-Dieter Schulzke, Matteo Serino, Herbert Tilg, Alastair Watson, and Jerry M. Wells. "Intestinal Permeability – a New Target for Disease Prevention and Therapy." BMC Gastroenterology. November 18, 2014. Accessed May 23, 2017. doi:10.1186/s12876-014-0189-7.

24. Drisko, J., B. Bischoff, M. Hall, and R. McCallum. "Treating Irritable Bowel Syndrome with a Food Elimination Diet Followed by Food Challenge and Probiotics." Journal of the American College of Nutrition. December 25, 2006. Accessed May 23, 2017. http://www.ncbi.nlm.nih.gov/pubmed/17229899.

25. Marchioni, R. M., and J. W. Birk. "Wheat-related Disorders Reviewed: Making a Grain of Sense." Expert Review of Gastroenterology & Hepatology. June 2015. Accessed May 23, 2017. doi:10.1586/17474124.2015.

26. Block, G., B. Patterson, and A. Subar. "Fruit, Vegetables, and Cancer Prevention: A Review of the Epidemiological Evidence." Nutrition and Cancer. Accessed May 23, 2017. doi:10.1080/01635589209514201.

27. Riboli, E., and T. Norat. "Epidemiologic Evidence of the Protective Effect of Fruit and Vegetables on Cancer Risk." The American Journal of Clinical Nutrition. September 2003. Accessed May 23, 2017. http://www.ncbi.nlm.nih.gov/pubmed/12936950.

28. Steinmetz, K. A., and J. D. Potter. "Vegetables, Fruit, and Cancer Prevention: A Review." Journal of the American Dietetic Association. October 1996. Accessed May 23, 2017. https://www.ncbi.nlm.nih.gov/pubmed/8841165.

29. Oude, L. M., J. M. Geleijnse, D. Kromhout, M. C. Ocké, and W. M. Verschuren. "Raw and Processed Fruit and Vegetable Consumption and 10-year Coronary Heart Disease Incidence in a Population-based Cohort Study in the Netherlands." PloS One. October 25, 2010. Accessed May 23, 2017. doi:10.1371/journal.pone.0013609.

30. Alonso, A., C. De, A. M. Martín-Arnau, J. De, J. A. Martínez, and M. A. Martínez-González. "Fruit and Vegetable Consumption Is Inversely Associated with Blood Pressure in a Mediterranean Population with a High Vegetable-fat Intake: The Seguimiento Universidad De Navarra (SUN) Study." The British Journal of Nutrition. August 2004. Accessed May 23, 2017. doi:10.1079/BJN20041196.

31. Wang, X., Y. Ouyang, J. Liu, M. Zhu, G. Zhao, W. Bao, and F. B. Hu. "Fruit and Vegetable Consumption and Mortality from All Causes, Cardiovascular Disease, and Cancer: Systematic Review and Dose-response Meta-analysis of Prospective Cohort Studies." British Medical Journal (Clinical Research Ed.). July 29, 2014. Accessed May 23, 2017. doi:10.1136/bmj.g4490.

32. O'Conner, Anahad. "How the Sugar Industry Shifted Blame to Fat." New York Times, September 12, 2016.

33. Simopoulos, A. P. "Omega-3 Fatty Acids in Inflammation and Autoimmune Diseases." Journal of the American College of Nutrition. December 21, 2002. Accessed May 23, 2017. https://www.ncbi.nlm.nih.gov/pubmed/12480795.

34. Patterson, E., R. Wall, G. F. Fitzgerald, R. P. Ross, and C. Stanton. "Health Implications of High Dietary Omega-6 Polyunsaturated Fatty Acids." Journal of Nutrition and Metabolism. 2012. Accessed May 23, 2017. doi:10.1155/2012/539426.

35. Siri-Tarino, Patty W., Qi Sun, and And Frank B Hu. "Patty W Siri-Tarino." The American Journal of Clinical Nutrition. January 13, 2010. Accessed May 06, 2017. doi:10.3945/ajcn.2009.27725.

36. Yang, PhD Quanhe. "Sugar Intake and Cardiovascular Diseases Mortality." JAMA Internal Medicine. April 01, 2014. Accessed May 26, 2017. doi:10.1001/jamainternmed.2013.13563.

37. Daley, Cynthia A., Amber Abbott, Patrick S. Doyle, Glenn A. Nader, and Stephanie Larson. "A Review of Fatty Acid Profiles and Antioxidant Content in Grass-fed and Grain-fed Beef." Nutrition Journal. 2010. Accessed May 23, 2017. doi:10.1186/1475-2891-9-10.

38.   Hunter, Beatrice T. "The Downside of Soybean Consumption." Nutrition Digest 38, no. 2 (2001). Accessed May 07, 2017. http://americannutritionassociation.org/newsletter/downside-soybean-consumption-0.

39.   Adeyemo, S.m., and A.a. Onilude. "Enzymatic Reduction of Anti-nutritional Factors in Fermenting Soybeans by Lactobacillus Plantarum Isolates from Fermenting Cereals." Nigerian Food Journal 31, no. 2 (May 10, 2015): 84-90. doi:10.1016/s0189-7241(15)30080-1.

40.   Kuhnlein, Harriet V., and Nancy J. Turner. Traditional Plant Foods of Canadian Indigenous Peoples: Nutrition, Botany, and Use. New York: Gordon and Breach, 1991.

41.   Nanri, Akiko, Tetsuya Mizoue, Kayo Kurotani, Atsushi Goto, Shino Oba, Mitsuhiko Noda, Norie Sawada, Shoichiro Tsugane, and For the Japan Public Health Center-Based Prospective Study Group. "Low-Carbohydrate Diet and Type 2 Diabetes Risk in Japanese Men and Women: The Japan Public Health Center-Based Prospective Study." PLoS ONE. February 19, 2015. Accessed May 23, 2017. doi:10.1371/journal.pone.0118377.

42.   Riebl, Shaun K., and Brenda M. Davy. "The Hydration Equation: Update on Water Balance and Cognitive Performance." ACSM's Health & Fitness Journal. November/December 2013. Accessed May 23, 2017. doi:10.1249/FIT.0b013e3182a9570f.

CHAPTER 4

1.   The Mayo, Clinic. "Chronic Stress Puts Your Health at Risk." Mayo Clinic. April 21, 2016. Accessed May 26, 2017. http://www.mayoclinic.org/healthy-lifestyle/stress-management/in-depth/stress/art-20046037.

2.   Publications, Harvard Health. "Understanding the Stress Response." Harvard Health. March 2011. Accessed May 26, 2017. http://www.health.harvard.edu/staying-healthy/understanding-the-stress-response.

3.   Wood, A. M., J. J. Froh, and A. W. Geraghty. "Gratitude and Well-being: A Review and Theoretical Integration." Clinical Psychology Review. November 2010. Accessed May 26, 2017. doi:10.1016/j.cpr.2010.03.005.

4.   Devlin, Hillary C., Jamil Zaki, Desmond C. Ong, and June Gruber. "Not As Good as You Think? Trait Positive Emotion Is Associated with Increased Self-Reported Empathy but Decreased Empathic Performance." PLOS ONE. October 29, 2014. Accessed May 26, 2017. doi:doi.org/10.1371/journal.pone.0110470.

5.   Redwine, L. S., B. L. Henry, M. A. Pung, K. Wilson, K. Chinh, B. Knight, S. Jain, T. Rutledge, B. Greenberg, A. Maisel, and P. J. Mills. "Pilot Randomized Study of a Gratitude Journaling Intervention on Heart Rate Variability and Inflammatory Biomarkers in Patients With Stage B Heart Failure." Psychosomatic Medicine. July/August 2016. Accessed May 26, 2017. doi:10.1097/PSY.0000000000000316.

6. Wood, Alex M., John Maltby, Raphael Gillett, P. Alex Linley, and Stephen Joseph. "The Role of Gratitude in the Development of Social Support, Stress, and Depression: Two Longitudinal Studies." Journal of Research in Personality 42, no. 4 (December 4, 2007): 854-71. Accessed May 06, 2017. doi:10.1016/j.jrp.2007.11.003.

7. Mills, Paul J., Laura Redwine, Kathleen Wilson, Meredith A. Pung, Kelly Chinh, Barry H. Greenberg, Ottar Lunde, Alan Maisel, Ajit Raisinghani, Alex Wood, and Deepak Chopra. "The Role of Gratitude in Spiritual Well-being in Asymptomatic Heart Failure Patients." Spirituality in Clinical Practice. March 2015. Accessed May 26, 2017. doi:10.1037/scp0000050.

8. Holt-Lunstad, J., T. B. Smith, and J. B. Layton. "Social Relationships and Mortality Risk: A Meta-analytic Review." PLoS Medicine. July 27, 2010. Accessed May 26, 2017. doi:10.1371/journal.pmed.1000316.

9. Valtorta, Nicole K., Mona Kanaan, Simon Gilbody, Sara Ronzi, and Barbara Hanratty. "Loneliness and Social Isolation as Risk Factors for Coronary Heart Disease and Stroke: Systematic Review and Meta-analysis of Longitudinal Observational Studies." Heart. March 15, 2016. Accessed May 26, 2017. doi:10.1136/heartjnl-2015-308790.

10. Robbins, John. Healthy at 100: The Scientifically Proven Secrets of the Worlds Healthiest and Longest-lived Peoples. Bath, England: Chivers Press, 2008.

11. Berkowitz, Gale. "UCLA Study On Friendship Among Women." CND: UCLA Study On Friendship Among Women. 2002. Accessed August 21, 2016. http://www.anapsid.org/cnd/gender/tendfend.html.

12. Kroenke, C. H., L. D. Kubzansky, E. S. Schernhammer, M. D. Holmes, and I. Kawachi. "Social Networks, Social Support, and Survival after Breast Cancer Diagnosis." Journal of Clinical Oncology : Official Journal of the American Society of Clinical Oncology. March 01, 2006. Accessed May 26, 2017. doi:10.1200/JCO.2005.04.2846.

13. Lucchetti, G., A. L. Lucchetti, and H. G. Koenig. "Impact of Spirituality/religiosity on Mortality: Comparison with Other Health Interventions." Explore (New York, N.Y.). July/August 2011. Accessed May 26, 2017. doi:10.1016/j.explore.2011.04.005.

14. Li, ScD Shanshan, Meir J. Stampher, David R. Williams, and Tyler J. VanderWeele. "Religious Service Attendance and Mortality Among Women." JAMA Internal Medicine. June 01, 2016. Accessed May 26, 2017. doi:10.1001/jamainternmed.2016.1615.

15. Bernardi, Luciano, Peter Sleight, Gabriele Bandinelli, Simone Cencetti, Lamberto Fattorini, Johanna Wdowczyc-Szulc, and Alfonso Lagi. "Effect of Rosary Prayer and Yoga Mantras on Autonomic Cardiovascular Rhythms: Comparative Study." British Medical Journal. December 22, 2001. Accessed May 26, 2017. https://www.ncbi.nlm.nih.gov/pmc/articles/PMC61046/.

16.	Kaliman, Perla, María Jesús Álvarez-López, Marta Cosín-Tomás, Melissa A. Rosenkranz, Antoine Lutz, and Richard J. Davidson. "Rapid Changes in Histone Deacetylases and Inflammatory Gene Expression in Expert Meditators." Psychoneuroendocrinology. February 2014. Accessed May 26, 2017. doi:10.1016/j.psyneuen.2013.11.004.

17.	Bellis, Rich. "Your Brain Has A." Fast Company. April 19, 2017. Accessed April 26, 2017. https://www.fastcompany.com/3059634/your-most-productive-self/your-brain-has-a-delete-button-heres-how-to-use-it.

18.	Abbasi, B., M. Kimiagar, K. Sadeghniiat, M. M. Shirazi, M. Hedayati, and B. Rashidkhani. "The Effect of Magnesium Supplementation on Primary Insomnia in Elderly: A Double-blind Placebo-controlled Clinical Trial." Journal of Research in Medical Sciences : The Official Journal of Isfahan University of Medical Sciences. December 17, 2012. Accessed May 26, 2017. https://www.ncbi.nlm.nih.gov/pubmed/23853635.

19.	Ngan, A., and R. Conduit. "A Double-blind, Placebo-controlled Investigation of the Effects of Passiflora Incarnata (passionflower) Herbal Tea on Subjective Sleep Quality." Phytotherapy Research : PTR. August 25, 2011. Accessed May 26, 2017. doi:10.1002/ptr.3400.

20.	Srivastava, Janmejai K., Eswar Shankar, and Sanjay Gupta. "Chamomile: A Herbal Medicine of the past with Bright Future." Molecular Medicine Reports. November 01, 2010. Accessed March 26, 2017. doi:10.3892/mmr.2010.377.

21.	Bent, Stephen, Amy Padula, Dan Moore, Michael Patterson, and Wolf Mehling. "Valerian for Sleep: A Systematic Review and Meta-Analysis." The American Journal of Medicine. December 2006. Accessed May 26, 2017. doi:10.1016/j.amjmed.2006.02.026.

22.	Chevalier, Gaétan, Stephen T. Sinatra, James L. Oschman, Karol Sokal, and Pawel Sokal. "Earthing: Health Implications of Reconnecting the Human Body to the Earth's Surface Electrons." Journal of Environmental and Public Health. 2012. Accessed May 26, 2017. doi:10.1155/2012/291541.

23.	Oschman, J. L. "Can Electrons Act as Antioxidants? A Review and Commentary." Journal of Alternative and Complementary Medicine (New York, N.Y.). November 13, 2007. Accessed May 26, 2017. doi:10.1089/acm.2007.7048.

24.	Chevalier, Gaétan, Stephen T. Sinatra, James L. Oschman, and Richard M. Delany. "Earthing (Grounding) the Human Body Reduces Blood Viscosity—a Major Factor in Cardiovascular Disease." Journal of Alternative and Complementary Medicine. February 19, 2013. Accessed May 26, 2017. doi:10.1089/acm.2011.0820.

25.	Sokal, K., and P. Sokal. "Earthing the Human Body Influences Physiologic Processes." Journal of Alternative and Complementary Medicine (New York, N.Y.). April 6, 2011. Accessed May 26, 2017. doi:10.1089/acm.2010.0687.

26.	Chevalier, Gaétan, Stephen T. Sinatra, James L. Oschman, Karol Sokal, and Pawel Sokal. "Earthing: Health Implications of Reconnecting the Human Body to the Earth's Surface Electrons." Journal of Environmental and Public Health. January 12, 2012. Accessed May 26, 2017. doi:10.1155/2012/291541.

27. Brown, Dick, Gaétan Chevalier, and Michael Hill. "Pilot Study on the Effect of Grounding on Delayed-Onset Muscle Soreness." Journal of Alternative and Complementary Medicine. March 16, 2010. Accessed May 26, 2017. doi:10.1089/acm.2009.0399.

28. Ghaly, M., and D. Teplitz. "The Biologic Effects of Grounding the Human Body during Sleep as Measured by Cortisol Levels and Subjective Reporting of Sleep, Pain, and Stress." Journal of Alternative and Complementary Medicine (New York, N.Y.). October 10, 2004. Accessed May 26, 2017. doi:10.1089/acm.2004.10.767.

29. Chevalier, Gaétan, and Stephen T. Sinatra. "Emotional Stress, Heart Rate Variability, Grounding, and Improved Autonomic Tone: Clinical Applications." Integrative Medicine: A Clinical Journal 10, no. 3 (June/July 2011). Accessed April 04, 2017. http://imjournal.com/pdfarticles/IMCJ10_3_p16_24chevalier.pdf.

30. Berg, Magdalena M.H.E. Van Den, Jolanda Maas, Rianne Muller, Anoek Braun, Wendy Kaandorp, René Van Lien, Mireille N.M. Van Poppel, Willem Van Mechelen, and Agnes E. Van Den Berg. "Autonomic Nervous System Responses to Viewing Green and Built Settings: Differentiating Between Sympathetic and Parasympathetic Activity." International Journal of Environmental Research and Public Health. December 12, 2015. Accessed May 26, 2017. doi:https://www.ncbi.nlm.nih.gov/pmc/articles/PMC4690962/.

31. Beyer, Kirsten M. M., Andrea Kaltenbach, Aniko Szabo, Sandra Bogar, F. Javier Nieto, and Kristen M. Malecki. "Exposure to Neighborhood Green Space and Mental Health: Evidence from the Survey of the Health of Wisconsin." International Journal of Environmental Research and Public Health. March 21, 2014. Accessed May 26, 2017. doi:10.3390/ijerph110303453.

32. Detweiler, Mark B., Taral Sharma, Jonna G. Detweiler, Pamela F. Murphy, Sandra Lane, Jack Carman, Amara S. Chudhary, Mary H. Halling, and Kye Y. Kim. "What Is the Evidence to Support the Use of Therapeutic Gardens for the Elderly?" Psychiatry Investigation. June 9, 2012. Accessed May 26, 2017. doi:10.4306/pi.2012.9.2.100.

33. Mishra, Badri N. "Secret of Eternal Youth; Teaching from the Centenarian Hot Spots ("Blue Zones")." Indian Journal of Community Medicine : Official Publication of Indian Association of Preventive & Social Medicine. October 2009. Accessed May 26, 2017. doi:10.4103/0970-0218.58380.

34. Kawata, Tomoyuki, A. Li, ARi Itoh-nakadai, and H. Suzuki. "Effect of Forest Bathing on Sleep and Physical Activity." Reserachgate.net. January 2013. Accessed May 05, 2017. https://www.researchgate.net/publication/288111347_Effect_of_forest_bathing_on_sleep_and_physical_activity.

35. King, D. E., 3. R. Mainous, M. E. Geesey, and R. F. Woolson. "Dietary Magnesium and C-reactive Protein Levels." Journal of the American College of Nutrition. June 2005. Accessed June 16, 2017. https://www.ncbi.nlm.nih.gov/pubmed/15930481.

36. Proksch, E., H. P. Nissen, M. Bremgartner, and C. Urquhart. "Bathing in a Magnesium-rich Dead Sea Salt Solution Improves Skin Barrier Function, Enhances Skin Hydration, and Reduces Inflammation in Atopic Dry Skin." International Journal of Dermatology. February 2005. Accessed May 29, 2017. doi:10.1111/j.1365-4632.2005.02079.x.

37. Sukenik, S., D. Flusser, S. Codish, and M. Abu-Shakra. "Balneotherapy at the Dead Sea Area for Knee Osteoarthritis." The Israel Medical Association Journal : IMAJ. October 1999. Accessed May 29, 2017. https://www.ncbi.nlm.nih.gov/pubmed/10731301.

38. Stuckey, Heather L., and Jeremy Nobel. "The Connection Between Art, Healing, and Public Health: A Review of Current Literature." American Journal of Public Health. February 2010. Accessed May 29, 2017. doi:10.2105/AJPH.2008.156497.

39. Mackay, Alison M., Robert Buckingham, Raymond S. Schwartz, Suzanne Hodgkinson, Roy G. Beran, and Dennis J. Cordato. "The Effect of Biofeedback as a Psychological Intervention in Multiple Sclerosis: A Randomized Controlled Study." International Journal of MS Care. May/June 2015. Accessed May 29, 2017. doi:10.7224/1537-2073.2014-006.

CHAPTER 5

1. NTP. "About NTP." National Institute of Environmental Health Sciences. Accessed May 29, 2017. https://ntp.niehs.nih.gov/about/index.html.

2. Andrews, David, Ph.D., and Richard Wiles. Off the Books: Industry's Secret Chemicals. Environmental Working Group, 2009. http://www.ewg.org/sites/default/files/report/secret-chemicals.pdf.

3. Environmental Working Group. "Body Burden: The Pollution in Newborns." EWG. July 14, 2005. Accessed May 29, 2017. http://www.ewg.org/research/body-burden-pollution-newborns.

4. DellaValle, Curt. "The Pollution in People." EWG. June 14, 2016. Accessed May 29, 2017. http://www.ewg.org/research/pollution-people.

5. Coster, Sam De, and Nicolas Van Larebeke. "Endocrine-Disrupting Chemicals: Associated Disorders and Mechanisms of Action." Journal of Environmental and Public Health. 2012. Accessed May 29, 2017. doi:10.1155/2012/713696.

6. Diamanti-Kandarakis, Evanthia, Jean-Pierre Bourguignon, Linda C. Giudice, Russ Hauser, Gail S. Prins, Ana M. Soto, R. Thomas Zoeller, and Andrea C. Gore. "Endocrine-Disrupting Chemicals: An Endocrine Society Scientific Statement." Endocrine Reviews. June 2009. Accessed May 29, 2017. doi:10.1210/er.2009-0002.

7. Qui, Wenhui. "Actions of Bisphenol a and Bisphenol S on the Reproductive Neuroendocrine System During Early Development in Zebrafish - Journals - NCBI." National Center for Biotechnology Information. December 10, 2015. Accessed May 29, 2017. doi:10.1210/en.2015-1785.

8.   Chen, Mei, Chi-Hsuan Chang, Lin Tao, and Chensheng Lu. "Residential Exposure to Pesticide During Childhood and Childhood Cancers: A Meta-Analysis." Pediatrics. September 01, 2015. Accessed May 29, 2017. http://pediatrics.aappublications.org/content/early/2015/09/08/peds.2015-0006?sid=6f4d081e-f317-4bdc-8ac6-8c6b9d6d42df.

9.   Kamel, Freya, and Jane A. Hoppin. "Association of Pesticide Exposure with Neurologic Dysfunction and Disease." Environmental Health Perspectives. June 2004. Accessed May 29, 2017. doi:10.1289/ehp.7135.

10. Grant, D. M. "Detoxification Pathways in the Liver." Journal of Inherited Metabolic Disease. 1991. Accessed May 29, 2017. https://www.ncbi.nlm.nih.gov/pubmed/1749210.

11. Watzl, B. "Anti-inflammatory Effects of Plant-based Foods and of Their Constituents." International Journal for Vitamin and Nutrition Research. Internationale Zeitschrift Fur Vitamin- Und Ernahrungsforschung. Journal International De Vitaminologie Et De Nutrition. December 2008. Accessed May 29, 2017. doi:10.1024/0300-9831.78.6.293.

12. Gimeno-García, E., V. Andreu, and R. Boluda. "Heavy Metals Incidence in the Application of Inorganic Fertilizers and Pesticides to Rice Farming Soils." Environmental Pollution (Barking, Essex : 1987). 1996. Accessed May 29, 2017. https://www.ncbi.nlm.nih.gov/pubmed/15091407.

13. Mnif, Wissem, Aziza Ibn Hadj Hassine, Aicha Bouaziz, Aghleb Bartegi, Olivier Thomas, and Benoit Roig. "Effect of Endocrine Disruptor Pesticides: A Review." International Journal of Environmental Research and Public Health. June 08, 2011. Accessed May 29, 2017. doi:10.3390/ijerph8062265.

14. Buettner, Dan. The Blue Zones: 9 Lessons for Living Longer from the People Who've Lived the Longest. Washington, D.C.: National Geographic, 2012.

15. Environmental Working Group. "National Drinking Water Database." Environmental Working Group. December 2009. Accessed May 29, 2017. http://www.ewg.org/tap-water/.

16. Tchounwou, Paul B., Clement G. Yedjou, Anita K. Patlolla, and Dwayne J. Sutton. "Heavy Metals Toxicity and the Environment." EXS. August 26, 2012. Accessed May 29, 2017. doi:10.1007/978-3-7643-8340-4_6.

17. Grandjean, Philippe, and Phillip Landrigan. "Neurobehavioural Effects of Developmental Toxicity." Thelancet.com. March 14, 2014. doi:http://dx.doi.org/10.1016/S1474-4422(13)70278-3.

18. Environmental Working Group. "Contaminants of Emerging Concern including Pharmaceuticals and Personal Care Products." EPA. September 27, 2016. Accessed May 29, 2017. https://www.epa.gov/wqc/contaminants-emerging-concern-including-pharmaceuticals-and-personal-care-products.

19. Snyder, Shane A. "Occurrence of Pharmaceuticals in U.S. Drinking Water." ACS Symposium Series. November 02, 2010. Accessed May 29, 2017. doi:10.1021/bk-2010-1048.ch003.

20. Environmental Working Group. "EWG's Consumer Guide to Seafood." EWG. September 18, 2014. Accessed May 29, 2017. http://www.ewg.org/research/ewgs-good-seafood-guide.

21. "Endocrine Disruptors." National Institute of Environmental Health Sciences. Accessed May 29, 2017. https://www.niehs.nih.gov/health/topics/agents/endocrine/.

22. Center for Food Safety and Applied Nutrition. "Potential Contaminants - Lead in Cosmetics." U S Food and Drug Administration Home Page. Accessed May 29, 2017. https://www.fda.gov/cosmetics/productsingredients/potentialcontaminants/ucm388820.htm.

23. Potera, Carol. "INDOOR AIR QUALITY: Scented Products Emit a Bouquet of VOCs." Environmental Health Perspectives. January 2011. Accessed May 29, 2017. doi:10.1289/ehp.119-a16.

24. Sunscreens, EWG's 2017 Guide to. "EWG's 2017 Guide to Safer Sunscreens." EWG. Accessed May 29, 2017. http://www.ewg.org/sunscreen/report/the-trouble-with-sunscreen-chemicals/.

25. Zock, Jan-Paul, Estel Plana, Deborah Jarvis, Josep M. Antó, Hans Kromhout, Susan M. Kennedy, Nino Künzli, Simona Villani, Mario Olivieri, Kjell Torén, Katja Radon, Jordi Sunyer, Anna Dahlman-Hoglund, Dan Norbäck, and Manolis Kogevinas. "The Use of Household Cleaning Sprays and Adult Asthma: An International Longitudinal Study." American Journal of Respiratory and Critical Care Medicine. October 15, 2007. Accessed May 29, 2017. doi:10.1164/rccm.200612-1793OC.

26. Dumas, Orianne, Carole Donnay, Dick J J Heederik, Michel Héry, Dominique Choudat, Francine Kauffmann, and Nicole Le Moual. "Occupational Exposure to Cleaning Products and Asthma in Hospital Workers." Occup Environ Med. December 01, 2012. Accessed May 29, 2017. doi:10.1136/oemed-2012-100826.

27. U.s. Epa Federal Facilities Restoration And Reuse Office. "United States Office of Solid Waste and EPA 505 -F -1 4-01 1 Environmental Protection Agency Emergency Response (5106P) January 2014. Technical Fact Sheet–1,4 -Dioxane." Technical Fact Sheet – 1,4-Dioxane, January 14, 2014. Accessed May 27, 2017. https://www.epa.gov/sites/production/files/2014-03/documents/ffrro_factsheet_contaminant_14-dioxane_january2014_final.pdf.

28. Environmental Working Group. "Cleaning Supplies and Your Health." EWG. Accessed May 29, 2017. http://www.ewg.org/guides/cleaners/content/cleaners_and_health.

29. Silent Spring. "Chemicals and Breast Cancer." Silent Spring Institute. July 30, 2014. Accessed May 29, 2017. http://silentspring.org/research-area/chemicals-and-breast-cancer.

30. Farrow, A., H. Taylor, K. Northstone, and J. Golding. "Symptoms of Mothers and Infants Related to Total Volatile Organic Compounds in Household Products." Archives of Environmental Health. October 2003. Accessed May 29, 2017. doi:10.3200/AEOH.58.10.633-641.

31. Mehta, Amar J., Martin Adam, Emmanuel Schaffner, Jean-Claude Barthélémy, David Carballo, Jean-Michel Gaspoz, Thierry Rochat, Christian Schindler, Joel Schwartz, Jan-Paul Zock, Nino Künzli, Nicole Probst-Hensch, and SAPALDIA Team. "Heart Rate Variability in Association with Frequent Use of Household Sprays and Scented Products in SAPALDIA." Environmental Health Perspectives. April 22, 2012. Accessed May 29, 2017. doi:10.1289/ehp.1104567.

32. Jacobson, Joseph L., and Sandra W. Jacobson. "Intellectual Impairment in Children Exposed to Polychlorinated Biphenyls in Utero — NEJM." New England Journal of Medicine. December 12, 1996. Accessed May 29, 2017. doi:10.1056/NEJM199609123351104.

33. Zhang, Yawei, Grace L. Guo, Xuesong Han, Cairong Zhu, Briseis A. Kilfoy, Yong Zhu, Peter Boyle, and Tongzhang Zheng. "Do Polybrominated Diphenyl Ethers (PBDEs) Increase the Risk of Thyroid Cancer?" Bioscience Hypotheses. 2008. Accessed May 29, 2017. doi:10.1016/j.bihy.2008.06.003.

34. "Electromagnetic Fields and Public Health: Mobile Phones." World Health Organization. October 2014. Accessed May 29, 2017. http://www.who.int/mediacentre/factsheets/fs193/en/.

35. Gorpinchenko, Igor, Oleg Nikitin, Oleg Banyra, and Alexander Shulyak. "The Influence of Direct Mobile Phone Radiation on Sperm Quality." Central European Journal of Urology. April 17, 2014. Accessed May 29, 2017. doi:10.5173/ceju.2014.01.art14.

36. Roggeveen, Suzanne, Jim Van Os, Wolfgang Viechtbauer, and Richel Lousberg. "EEG Changes Due to Experimentally Induced 3G Mobile Phone Radiation." PLoS ONE. 2015. Accessed May 29, 2017. doi:10.1371/journal.pone.0129496.

37. Mahmoudabadi, Fatemeh Shamsi, Saeideh Ziaei, Mohammad Firoozabadi, and Anoshirvan Kazemnejad. "Use of Mobile Phone during Pregnancy and the Risk of Spontaneous Abortion." Journal of Environmental Health Science and Engineering. April 21, 2015. Accessed May 29, 2017. doi:10.1186/s40201-015-0193-z.

38. United States Environmental Protection Agency. Basis for Educational Recommendations on Reducing Childhood Lead Exposure. Bibliogov, 2012. Accessed May 29, 2017. https://www.epa.gov/sites/production/files/documents/reduc_pb.pdf.

39. Genuis, S. J., D. Birkholz, I. Rodushkin, and S. Beesoon. "Blood, Urine, and Sweat (BUS) Study: Monitoring and Elimination of Bioaccumulated Toxic Elements." Archives of Environmental Contamination and Toxicology. November 06, 2010. Accessed May 29, 2017. doi:10.1007/s00244-010-9611-5.

40. Genuis, S. J., S. Beesoon, D. Birkholz, and R. A. Lobo. "Human Excretion of Bisphenol A: Blood, Urine, and Sweat (BUS) Study." Journal of Environmental and Public Health. December 27, 2011. Accessed May 29, 2017. doi:10.1155/2012/185731.

41. Sears, Margaret E., Kathleen J. Kerr, and Riina I. Bray. "Arsenic, Cadmium, Lead, and Mercury in Sweat: A Systematic Review." Journal of Environmental and Public Health. February 22, 2012. Accessed May 29, 2017. doi:10.1155/2012/184745.

42. Sapolsky, Robert M. "Why Stress Is Bad for Your Brain." Science 273, no. 5276, 749-50. doi:10.1126/science.273.5276.749.

CHAPTER 6

1. Sender, Ron, Shai Fuchs, and Ron Milo. "Revised Estimates for the Number of Human and Bacteria Cells in the Body." PLoS Biology. August 2016. Accessed June 02, 2017. doi:10.1371/journal.pbio.1002533.

2. Galland, Leo. "The Gut Microbiome and the Brain." Journal of Medicinal Food. December 01, 2014. Accessed June 02, 2017. doi:10.1089/jmf.2014.7000.

3. Zheng, Gen, Shu-Pei Wu, Yongjun Hu, David E. Smith, John W. Wiley, and Shuangsong Hong. "Corticosterone Mediates Stress-related Increased Intestinal Permeability in a Region-specific Manner." Neurogastroenterology and Motility : The Official Journal of the European Gastrointestinal Motility Society. February 2013. Accessed June 02, 2017. doi:10.1111/nmo.12066.

4. Cogan, T. A., A. O. Thomas, L. E N Rees, A. H. Taylor, M. A. Jepson, P. H. Williams, J. Ketley, and T. J. Humphrey. "Norepinephrine Increases the Pathogenic Potential of Campylobacter Jejuni." Gut. August 2007. Accessed June 04, 2017. doi:10.1136/gut.2006.114926.

5. Kelly, J. R., P. J. Kennedy, J. F. Cryan, T. G. Dinan, G. Clarke, and N. P. Hyland. "Breaking down the Barriers: The Gut Microbiome, Intestinal Permeability and Stress-related Psychiatric Disorders." Frontiers in Cellular Neuroscience. October 14, 2015. Accessed June 04, 2017. doi:10.3389/fncel.2015.00392.

6. Cogan, T. A., A. O. Thomas, L. E N Rees, A. H. Taylor, M. A. Jepson, P. H. Williams, J. Ketley, and T. J. Humphrey. "Norepinephrine Increases the Pathogenic Potential of Campylobacter Jejuni." Gut. August 2007. Accessed June 02, 2017. doi:10.1136/gut.2006.114926.

7. Rakoff-Nahoum, Seth. "Why Cancer and Inflammation?" The Yale Journal of Biology and Medicine. October 2007. Accessed June 02, 2017. https://www.ncbi.nlm.nih.gov/pmc/articles/PMC1994795/.

8. Slavich, George M., and Michael R. Irwin. "From Stress to Inflammation and Major Depressive Disorder: A Social Signal Transduction Theory of Depression." Psychological Bulletin. January 13, 2014. Accessed June 02, 2017. doi:10.1037/a0035302.

9. Kelly, J. R., P. J. Kennedy, J. F. Cryan, T. G. Dinan, G. Clarke, and N. P. Hyland. "Breaking down the Barriers: The Gut Microbiome, Intestinal Permeability and Stress-related Psychiatric Disorders." Frontiers in Cellular Neuroscience. October 14, 2015. Accessed June 02, 2017. doi:10.3389/fncel.2015.00392.

10. Cryan, J. F., and T. G. Dinan. "Mind-altering Microorganisms: The Impact of the Gut Microbiota on Brain and Behaviour." Nature Reviews. Neuroscience. September 12, 2012. Accessed June 02, 2017. doi:10.1038/nrn3346.

11. Fadgyas-Stanculete, M., A. M. Buga, A. Popa-Wagner, and D. L. Dumitrascu. "The Relationship between Irritable Bowel Syndrome and Psychiatric Disorders: From Molecular Changes to Clinical Manifestations." Journal of Molecular Psychiatry. June 27, 2014. Accessed June 02, 2017. doi:10.1186/2049-9256-2-4.

12. Bowe, Whitney P., and Alan C. Logan. "Acne Vulgaris, Probiotics and the Gut-brain-skin Axis - Back to the Future?" Gut Pathogens. January 31, 2011. Accessed June 02, 2017. doi:10.1186/1757-4749-3-1.

13. Morris, G., M. Berk, A. F. Carvalho, J. R. Caso, Y. Sanz, and M. Maes. "The Role of Microbiota and Intestinal Permeability in the Pathophysiology of Autoimmune and Neuroimmune Processes with an Emphasis on Inflammatory Bowel Disease Type I Diabetes and Chronic Fatigue Syndrome." Current Pharmaceutical Design. 2016. Accessed June 02, 2017. https://www.ncbi.nlm.nih.gov/pubmed/27634186.

14. Homayouni-Rad, A., A. R. Soroush, L. Khalili, L. Norouzi-Panahi, Z. Kasaie, and H. S. Ejtahed. "Diabetes Management by Probiotics: Current Knowledge and Future Pespective." International Journal for Vitamin and Nutrition Research. Internationale Zeitschrift Fur Vitamin- Und Ernahrungsforschung. Journal International De Vitaminologie Et De Nutrition. Accessed June 02, 2017. doi:10.1024/0300-9831/a000273.

15. De, N. M., C. G. Giezenaar, J. M. Rovers, B. J. Witteman, M. G. Smits, and S. Van. "The Effects of the Multispecies Probiotic Mixture Ecologic®Barrier on Migraine: Results of an Open-label Pilot Study." Beneficial Microbes. Accessed June 02, 2017. doi:10.3920/BM2015.0003.

16. Morris, G., M. Berk, A. F. Carvalho, J. R. Caso, Y. Sanz, and M. Maes. "The Role of Microbiota and Intestinal Permeability in the Pathophysiology of Autoimmune and Neuroimmune Processes with an Emphasis on Inflammatory Bowel Disease Type I Diabetes and Chronic Fatigue Syndrome." Current Pharmaceutical Design. 2006. Accessed June 02, 2017. https://www.ncbi.nlm.nih.gov/pubmed/27634186.

17. Tremellen, K., and K. Pearce. "Dysbiosis of Gut Microbiota (DOGMA)--a Novel Theory for the Development of Polycystic Ovarian Syndrome." Medical Hypotheses. April 27, 2012. Accessed June 02, 2017. doi:10.1016/j.mehy.2012.04.016.

18. Rapin, Jean Robert, and Nicolas Wiernsperger. "Possible Links between Intestinal Permeablity and Food Processing: A Potential Therapeutic Niche for Glutamine." Clinics. June 2010. Accessed June 02, 2017. doi:10.1590/S1807-59322010000600012.

19. Visser, Jeroen, Jan Rozing, Anna Sapone, Karen Lammers, and Alessio Fasano. "Tight Junctions, Intestinal Permeability, and Autoimmunity Celiac Disease and Type I Diabetes Paradigms." Annals of the New York Academy of Sciences. May 2009. Accessed June 02, 2017. doi:10.1111/j.1749-6632.2009.04037.x.

20. Sapone, A., J. C. Bai, C. Ciacci, J. Dolinsek, P. H. Green, M. Hadjivassiliou, K. Kaukinen, K. Rostami, D. S. Sanders, M. Schumann, R. Ullrich, D. Villalta, U. Volta, C. Catassi, and A. Fasano. "Spectrum of Gluten-related Disorders: Consensus on New Nomenclature and Classification." BMC Medicine. February 07, 2012. Accessed June 02, 2017. doi:10.1186/1741-7015-10-13.

21. Catassi, Carlo, Julio C. Bai, Bruno Bonaz, Gerd Bouma, Antonio Calabrò, Antonio Carroccio, Gemma Castillejo, Carolina Ciacci, Fernanda Cristofori, Jernej Dolinsek, Ruggiero Francavilla, Luca Elli, Peter Green, Wolfgang Holtmeier, Peter Koehler, Sibylle Koletzko, Christof Meinhold, David Sanders, Michael Schumann, Detlef Schuppan, Reiner Ullrich, Andreas Vécsei, Umberto Volta, Victor Zevallos, Anna Sapone, and Alessio Fasano. "Non-Celiac Gluten Sensitivity: The New Frontier of Gluten Related Disorders." Nutrients. October 2013. Accessed June 02, 2017. doi:10.3390/nu5103839.

22. Tulstrup, Monica Vera-Lise, Ellen Gerd Christensen, Vera Carvalho, Caroline Linninge, Siv Ahrné, Ole Højberg, Tine Rask Licht, and Martin Iain Bahl. "Antibiotic Treatment Affects Intestinal Permeability and Gut Microbial Composition in Wistar Rats Dependent on Antibiotic Class." PLoS ONE. December 21, 2015. Accessed June 02, 2017. doi:10.1371/journal.pone.0144854.

23. Bloomfield, SF, R. Stanwell-Smith, RWR Crevel, and J. Pickup. "Too Clean, or Not Too Clean: The Hygiene Hypothesis and Home Hygiene." Clinical and Experimental Allergy. April 2006. Accessed June 02, 2017. doi:10.1111/j.1365-2222.2006.02463.x.

24. Bjarnason, I., and K. Takeuchi. "Intestinal Permeability in the Pathogenesis of NSAID-induced Enteropathy." Journal of Gastroenterology. Accessed June 02, 2017. doi:10.1007/s00535-008-2266-6.

25. Buhner, S., C. Buning, J. Genschel, K. Kling, D. Herrmann, A. Dignass, I. Kuechler, S. Krueger, H. H. Schmidt, and H. Lochs. "Genetic Basis for Increased Intestinal Permeability in Families with Crohn's Disease: Role of CARD15 3020insC Mutation?" Gut. March 2006. Accessed June 02, 2017. doi:10.1136/gut.2005.065557.

26. Dukowicz, Andrew C., Brian E. Lacy, and Gary M. Levine. "Small Intestinal Bacterial Overgrowth: A Comprehensive Review." Gastroenterology & Hepatology. February 2007. Accessed June 02, 2017. https://www.ncbi.nlm.nih.gov/pmc/articles/PMC3099351/.

27. Makino, Hiroshi, Akira Kushiro, Eiji Ishikawa, Hiroyuki Kubota, Agata Gawad, Takafumi Sakai, Kenji Oishi, Rocio Martin, Kaouther Ben-Amor, Jan Knol, and Ryuichiro Tanaka. "Mother-to-Infant Transmission of Intestinal Bifidobacterial Strains Has an Impact on the Early Development of Vaginally Delivered Infant's Microbiota." PLOS ONE. Accessed June 02, 2017. doi:10.1371/journal.pone.0078331.

28. "Newborns Exposed to Dirt, Dander and Germs May Have Lower Allergy and Asthma Risk - 06/06/2014." Johns Hopkins Medicine, Based in Baltimore, Maryland. June 6, 2014. Accessed June 02, 2017. http://www.hopkinsmedicine.org/news/media/releases/newborns_exposed_to_dirt_dander_and_germs_may_have_lower_allergy_and_asthma_risk.

29. Skrovanek, Sonja, Katherine DiGuilio, Robert Bailey, William Huntington, Ryan Urbas, Barani Mayilvaganan, Giancarlo Mercogliano, and James M. Mullin. "Zinc and Gastrointestinal Disease." World Journal of Gastrointestinal Pathophysiology. November 15, 2014. Accessed June 02, 2017. doi:10.4291/wjgp.v5.i4.496.

30. Wang, Yizhong, Xiaolu Li, Ting Ge, Yongmei Xiao, Yang Liao, Yun Cui, Yucai Zhang, Wenzhe Ho, Guangjun Yu, and Ting Zhang. "Probiotics for Prevention and Treatment of Respiratory Tract Infections in Children: A Systematic Review and Meta-analysis of Randomized Controlled Trials." Medicine. August 2016. Accessed June 02, 2017. doi:10.1097/MD.0000000000004509.

31. Delzenne, N. M., A. M. Neyrinck, F. Bäckhed, and P. D. Cani. "Targeting Gut Microbiota in Obesity: Effects of Prebiotics and Probiotics." Nature Reviews. Endocrinology. August 09, 2011. Accessed June 02, 2017. doi:10.1038/nrendo.2011.126.

32. O'Neil, Jim. Antimicrobial Resistance: Tackling a Crisis for the Health and Wealth of Nations. United Kingdom: Review on Antimicrobial Resistance, 2014. Accessed May 27, 2017. https://amr-review.org/sites/default/files/AMR%20Review%20Paper%20-%20Tackling%20a%20crisis%20for%20the%20health%20and%20wealth%20of%20nations_1.pdf

33. Rennard, Barbara O., Ronald F. Ertl, Gail L. Gossman, Richard A. Robbins, and Stephen I. Rennard. "Chicken Soup Inhibits Neutrophil Chemotaxis In Vitro." CHEST Journal. October 01, 2000. Accessed June 02, 2017. doi:10.1378/chest.118.4.1150.

34. Tiralongo, E., R. A. Lea, S. S. Wee, M. M. Hanna, and L. R. Griffiths. "Randomised, Double Blind, Placebo-Controlled Trial of Echinacea Supplementation in Air Travellers." Evidence-based Complementary and Alternative Medicine : ECAM. 2012. Accessed June 02, 2017. doi:10.1155/2012/417267.

35. Tiralongo, Evelin, Shirley S. Wee, and Rodney A. Lea. "Elderberry Supplementation Reduces Cold Duration and Symptoms in Air-Travellers: A Randomized, Double-Blind Placebo-Controlled Clinical Trial." Nutrients. April 2016. Accessed June 02, 2017. doi:10.3390/nu8040182.

36. Kalemba, D., and A. Kunicka. "Antibacterial and Antifungal Properties of Essential Oils." Current Medicinal Chemistry. May 10, 2003. Accessed June 02, 2017. https://www.ncbi.nlm.nih.gov/pubmed/12678685.

37. Sadlon, A. E., and D. W. Lamson. "Immune-modifying and Antimicrobial Effects of Eucalyptus Oil and Simple Inhalation Devices." Alternative Medicine Review: A Journal of Clinical Therapeutic. April 2010. Accessed June 02, 2017. https://www.ncbi.nlm.nih.gov/pubmed/20359267.

38. Bayan, Leyla, Peir Hossain Koulivand, and Ali Gorji. "Garlic: A Review of Potential Therapeutic Effects." Avicenna Journal of Phytomedicine. 2014. Accessed June 02, 2017. https://www.ncbi.nlm.nih.gov/pmc/articles/PMC4103721/.

39. Bode, Ann M. "7: The Amazing and Mighty Ginger." In Herbal Medicine: Biomolecular and Clinical Aspects. 2nd ed. Boca Raton: CRC Press/Taylor & Francis, 2011.

40. Omar, Syed Haris. "Oleuropein in Olive and Its Pharmacological Effects." Scientia Pharmaceutica. 2010. Accessed June 02, 2017. doi:10.3797/scipharm.0912-18.

41.   Mathie, Robert T., Joyce Frye, and Peter Fisher. "Homeopathic Oscillococcinum®
      for Preventing and Treating Influenza and Influenza-like Illness." John Wiley and
      Sons, Ltd. January 28, 2015. Accessed June 02, 2017. doi:10.1002/14651858.CD001957.
      pub6.

42.   Ashraf, R., and N. P. Shah. "Immune System Stimulation by Probiotic
      Microorganisms." Critical Reviews in Food Science and Nutrition. Accessed June
      02, 2017. doi:10.1080/10408398.2011.619671.

43.   Moghadamtousi, Soheil Zorofchian, Habsah Abdul Kadir, Pouya Hassandarvish,
      Hassan Tajik, Sazaly Abubakar, and Keivan Zandi. "A Review on Antibacterial,
      Antiviral, and Antifungal Activity of Curcumin." BioMed Research International.
      2014. Accessed June 02, 2017. doi:10.1155/2014/186864.

44.   Ströhle, A., and A. Hahn. "[Vitamin C and Immune Function]." Medizinische
      Monatsschrift Fur Pharmazeuten. February 2009. Accessed June 02, 2017. https://
      www.ncbi.nlm.nih.gov/pubmed/19263912.

45.   Martineau, Adrian R., David A. Jolliffe, Richard L. Hooper, Lauren Greenberg,
      John F. Aloia, Peter Bergman, Gal Dubnov-Raz, Susanna Esposito, Davaasambuu
      Ganmaa, Adit A. Ginde, Emma C. Goodall, Cameron C. Grant, Christopher J.
      Griffiths, Wim Janssens, Ilkka Laaksi, Semira Manaseki-Holland, David Mauger,
      David R. Murdoch, Rachel Neale, Judy R. Rees, Steve Simpson, Iwona Stelmach,
      Geeta Trilok Kumar, Mitsuyoshi Urashima, and Carlos A. Camargo. "Vitamin
      D Supplementation to Prevent Acute Respiratory Tract Infections: Systematic
      Review and Meta-analysis of Individual Participant Data." British Medical Journal.
      February 15, 2017. Accessed June 02, 2017. doi:10.1136/bmj.i6583.

46.   Hemilä, Harri. "Zinc Lozenges May Shorten the Duration of Colds: A Systematic
      Review." The Open Respiratory Medicine Journal. June 23, 2011. Accessed June 02,
      2017. doi:10.2174/1874306401105010051.

47.   Vighi, G., F. Marcucci, L. Sensi, G. Di Cara, and F. Frati. "Allergy and the
      Gastrointestinal System." Clinical and Experimental Immunology. September 2008.
      Accessed June 10, 2017. doi:10.1111/j.1365-2249.2008.03713.x.

48.   Sarkar, Amar, Soili M. Lehto, Siobhán Harty, Timothy G. Dinan, John F. Cryan,
      and Philip W.J. Burnet. "Psychobiotics and the Manipulation of Bacteria–Gut–
      Brain Signals." Trends in Neurosciences. November 2016. Accessed June 02, 2017.
      doi:10.1016/j.tins.2016.09.002.

CHAPTER 7

1.   Jagadamma, S., R. Lal, and B.k. Rimal. "Effects of Topsoil Depth and Soil
      Amendments on Corn Yield and Properties of Two Alfisols in Central Ohio."
      Journal of Soil and Water Conservation 64, no. 1 (2009): 70-80. doi:10.2489/
      jswc.64.1.70.

2. Davis, Donald R., Melvin D. Epp, and Hugh D. Riordan. "Changes in USDA Food Composition Data for 43 Garden Crops, 1950 to 1999." Journal of the American College of Nutrition 23, no. 6 (December 2004): 669-82. doi:10.1080/07315724.200 4.10719409.

3. Santis, Stefania De, Elisabetta Cavalcanti, Mauro Mastronardi, Emilio Jirillo, and Marcello Chieppa. "Nutritional Keys for Intestinal Barrier Modulation." Frontiers in Immunology 6 (2015). doi:10.3389/fimmu.2015.00612.

4. Micronutrients, Macro Impact: The Story of Vitamins and a Hungry World. Basel, Switzerland: Sight and Life Press. Accessed March 5, 2017. http://www.sightandlife. org/fileadmin/data/Books/Micronutrients_Macro_Impact.pdf.

5. Iron Deficiency Anaemia Assessment Prevention and Control. World Health Organization. 15.

6. Abbaspour, Nazanin, Richard Hurrell, and Roya Kelishadi. "Review on Iron and Its Importance for Human Health." Journal of Research in Medical Sciences : The Official Journal of Isfahan University of Medical Sciences. February 2014. Accessed June 02, 2017. https://www.ncbi.nlm.nih.gov/pmc/articles/PMC3999603/.

7. "What Causes Anemia?" National Heart Lung and Blood Institute. May 18, 2012. Accessed June 02, 2017. https://www.nhlbi.nih.gov/health/health-topics/topics/ anemia/causes.

8. Jáuregui-Lobera, Ignacio. "Iron Deficiency and Cognitive Functions." Neuropsychiatric Disease and Treatment. 2014. Accessed June 02, 2017. doi:10.2147/ NDT.S72491.

9. Abbaspour, Nazanin, Richard Hurrell, and Roya Kelishadi. "Review on Iron and Its Importance for Human Health." Journal of Research in Medical Sciences : The Official Journal of Isfahan University of Medical Sciences. February 2014. Accessed June 02, 2017. https://www.ncbi.nlm.nih.gov/pmc/articles/PMC3999603/.

10. Jacobs, A., and G.M. Owen. "Effect of Gastric Juice on Iron Absorption in Patients with Gastric Atrophy." Gut 10 (1969): 488-90. Accessed March 27, 2017. https:// www.ncbi.nlm.nih.gov/pmc/articles/PMC1552937/pdf/gut00696-0082.pdf.

11. Schade, Stanley G., MD, Richard J. Cohen, MD, and Marcel E. Conrad, MD. "Effect of Hydrochloric Acid on Iron Absorption — NEJM." New England Journal of Medicine. Accessed June 04, 2017. doi:10.1056/NEJM196809262791302.

12. Hallberg, L. "Wheat Fiber, Phytates and Iron Absorption." Scandinavian Journal of Gastroenterology. Supplement. Accessed June 04, 2017. https://www.ncbi.nlm.nih. gov/pubmed/2820048.

13. Colleen Walsh, Harvard Staff Writer |, Anna Steinbock Harvard Correspondent |, Alvin Powell, Harvard Staff Writer |, and John Laidler Harvard Correspondent |. "A Genetic Cause for Iron Deficiency." Harvard Gazette. April 09, 2008. Accessed June 04, 2017. http://news.harvard.edu/gazette/ story/2008/04/a-genetic-cause-for-iron-deficiency/.

14. Friedman, A. J., A. Shander, S. R. Martin, R. K. Calabrese, M. E. Ashton, I. Lew, M. H. Seid, and L. T. Goodnough. "Iron Deficiency Anemia in Women: A Practical Guide to Detection, Diagnosis, and Treatment." Obstetrical & Gynecological Survey. May 2015. Accessed June 04, 2017. doi:10.1097/OGX.0000000000000172.

15. Hallberg, L., M. Brune, and L. Rossander. "The Role of Vitamin C in Iron Absorption." International Journal for Vitamin and Nutrition Research. Supplement = Internationale Zeitschrift Fur Vitamin- Und Ernahrungsforschung. Supplement. Accessed June 04, 2017. https://www.ncbi.nlm.nih.gov/pubmed/2507689.

16. Miller, Jeffery L. "Iron Deficiency Anemia: A Common and Curable Disease." Cold Spring Harbor Perspectives in Medicine. July 2013. Accessed June 04, 2017. doi:10.1101/cshperspect.a011866.

17. Geerligs, P. D., B. J. Brabin, and A. A. Omari. "Food Prepared in Iron Cooking Pots as an Intervention for Reducing Iron Deficiency Anaemia in Developing Countries: A Systematic Review." Journal of Human Nutrition and Dietetics : The Official Journal of the British Dietetic Association. August 2003. Accessed June 04, 2017. https://www.ncbi.nlm.nih.gov/pubmed/12859709.

18. "Pernicious Anemia." National Center for Biotechnology Information. June 11, 2014. Accessed June 04, 2017. https://www.ncbi.nlm.nih.gov/pubmedhealth/PMH0063030/.

19. Bissoli, L., V. Di, A. Ballarin, R. Mandragona, R. Trespidi, G. Brocco, B. Caruso, O. Bosello, and M. Zamboni. "Effect of Vegetarian Diet on Homocysteine Levels." Annals of Nutrition & Metabolism. Accessed June 04, 2017. doi:57644.

20. McBride, Judy. "Related Topics." B12 Deficiency May Be More Widespread Than Thought : USDA ARS. August 02, 2000. Accessed June 04, 2017. https://www.ars.usda.gov/news-events/news/research-news/2000/b12-deficiency-may-be-more-widespread-than-thought/.

21. Dukowicz, Andrew C., Brian E. Lacy, and Gary M. Levine. "Small Intestinal Bacterial Overgrowth: A Comprehensive Review." Gastroenterology & Hepatology. February 03, 2007. Accessed June 04, 2017. https://www.ncbi.nlm.nih.gov/pmc/articles/PMC3099351/.

22. Oh, Robert C., and David L. Brown. "Vitamin B12 Deficiency." American Family Physician. March 01, 2003. Accessed June 04, 2017. http://www.aafp.org/afp/2003/0301/p979.html.

23. "Vitamin Deficiency Anemia." Mayo Clinic. November 09, 2016. Accessed June 04, 2017. http://www.mayoclinic.org/diseases-conditions/vitamin-deficiency-anemia/symptoms-causes/dxc-20265323.

24. O'Leary, Fiona, and Samir Samman. "Vitamin B12 in Health and Disease." Nutrients. March 2010. Accessed June 04, 2017. doi:10.3390/nu2030299.

25. Handy, Diane E., Rita Castro, and Joseph Loscalzo. "Epigenetic Modifications: Basic Mechanisms and Role in Cardiovascular Disease." Circulation. May 17, 2011. Accessed June 04, 2017. doi:10.1161/CIRCULATIONAHA.110.956839.

26. "Does Vitamin D Play a Role in Your Health Condition?" Vitamin D Council. Accessed June 04, 2017. https://www.vitamindcouncil.org/health-conditions/.

27. Kennel, Kurt A., Matthew T. Drake, and Daniel L. Hurley. "Vitamin D Deficiency in Adults: When to Test and How to Treat." Mayo Clinic Proceedings. August 2010. Accessed June 04, 2017. doi:10.4065/mcp.2010.0138.

28. Nair, Rathish, and Arun Maseeh. "Vitamin D: The "sunshine" Vitamin." Journal of Pharmacology & Pharmacotherapeutics. 2012. Accessed June 04, 2017. doi:10.4103/0976-500X.95506.

29. "Why Does the Vitamin D Council Recommend 5,000 IU/day?" Vitamin D Council. Accessed June 04, 2017. https://www.vitamindcouncil.org/why-does-the-vitamin-d-council-recommend-5000-iuday/.

30. Holick, Michael F. "Vitamin D and Sunlight: Strategies for Cancer Prevention and Other Health Benefits." Clinical Journal of the American Society of Nephrology. Accessed May 27, 2017. doi:10.2215/CJN.01350308.

31. "Hypothyroidism - National Library of Medicine - PubMed Health." National Center for Biotechnology Information. Accessed June 04, 2017. https://www.ncbi.nlm.nih.gov/pubmedhealth/PMHT0022776/.

32. Kawicka, A., and B. Regulska-llow. "[Metabolic Disorders and Nutritional Status in Autoimmune Thyroid Diseases]." Postepy Higieny I Medycyny Doswiadczalnej (Online). January 02, 2015. Accessed June 04, 2017. doi:10.5604/17322693.1136383.

33. Ryan, Karen K. "11: Stress and Metabolic Disease." In Sociality, Hierarchy, Health: Comparative Biodemography: A Collection of Papers. Washington, DC: National Academies Press, 2014.

34. "Candidiasis - National Library of Medicine - PubMed Health." National Center for Biotechnology Information. Accessed June 04, 2017. https://www.ncbi.nlm.nih.gov/pubmedhealth/PMHT0024526/.

35. "Mercury in Dental Amalgam." EPA. December 15, 2016. Accessed June 04, 2017. https://www.epa.gov/mercury/mercury-dental-amalgam.

CHAPTER 8

1. Bradberry, Travis. "Multitasking Damages Your Brain And Career, New Studies Suggest." Forbes, October 08, 2014. Accessed June 04, 2017. https://www.forbes.com/forbes/welcome/?toURL=https%3A%2F%2Fwww.forbes.com%2Fsites%2Ftravisbradberry%2F2014%2F10%2F08%2Fmultitasking-damages-your-brain-and-career-new-studies-suggest%2F&refURL=&referrer=#7e4b8f4856ee.

2. Flaxman, Greg, Ph.D., and Lisa Flook, Ph.D. "Brief Summary of Mindfulness Research." Mindfulness Awareness Research Center UCLA Health. Accessed June 04, 2017. http://marc.ucla.edu/workfiles/pdfs/MARC-mindfulness-research-summary.pdf.

3. Whitebird, Robin R., Mary Jo Kreitzer, and Patrick J. O'Connor. "Mindfulness-Based Stress Reduction and Diabetes." Diabetes Spectrum : A Publication of the American Diabetes Association. September 21, 2009. Accessed June 04, 2017. doi:10.2337/diaspect.22.4.226.

4. Li, A. W., and C. A. Goldsmith. "The Effects of Yoga on Anxiety and Stress." Alternative Medicine Review : A Journal of Clinical Therapeutic. March 2012. Accessed June 04, 2017. https://www.ncbi.nlm.nih.gov/pubmed/22502620.

5. Streeter, Chris C., Theodore H. Whitfield, Liz Owen, Tasha Rein, Surya K. Karri, Aleksandra Yakhkind, Ruth Perlmutter, Andrew Prescot, Perry F. Renshaw, Domenic A. Ciraulo, and J. Eric Jensen. "Effects of Yoga Versus Walking on Mood, Anxiety, and Brain GABA Levels: A Randomized Controlled MRS Study." Journal of Alternative and Complementary Medicine. November 2010. Accessed June 04, 2017. doi:10.1089/acm.2010.0007.

6. Xiong, Xingjiang, Pengqian Wang, Xiaoke Li, and Yuqing Zhang. "Qigong for Hypertension: A Systematic Review." Medicine (Baltimore). January 2015. Accessed June 04, 2017. doi:10.1097/MD.0000000000000352.

7. Lee, M. S., M. H. Pittler, and E. Ernst. "Internal Qigong for Pain Conditions: A Systematic Review." The Journal of Pain : Official Journal of the American Pain Society. June 25, 2009. Accessed June 04, 2017. doi:10.1016/j.jpain.2009.03.009.

8. Wang, Chong-Wen, Celia HY Chan, Rainbow TH Ho, Jessie SM Chan, Siu-Man Ng, and Cecilia LW Chan. "Managing Stress and Anxiety through Qigong Exercise in Healthy Adults: A Systematic Review and Meta-analysis of Randomized Controlled Trials." BMC Complementary and Alternative Medicine. 2014. Accessed June 04, 2017. doi:10.1186/1472-6882-14-8.

9. Rosenbaum, Mark S., and Jane Van De Velde. "The Effects of Yoga, Massage, and Reiki on Patient Well-Being at a Cancer Resource Center." Clinical Journal of Oncology Nursing. June 01, 2016. Accessed June 04, 2017. doi:10.1188/16.CJON.E77-E81.

10. Thrane, Susan E., PhD, MSN, RN, Scott H. Maurer, and Dianxu Ren. "Reiki Therapy for Symptom Management in Children Receiving Palliative Care: A Pilot Study." American Journal of Hospice and Palliative Medicine®. February 07, 2016. Accessed June 04, 2017. doi:10.1177/1049909116630973.

11. "Food Poisoning." University of Maryland Medical Center. Accessed June 04, 2017. http://www.umm.edu/health/medical/altmed/condition/food-poisoning.

12. Hilton, E., P. Kolakowski, C. Singer, and M. Smith. "Efficacy of Lactobacillus GG as a Diarrheal Preventive in Travelers." Journal of Travel Medicine. March 01, 1997. Accessed June 04, 2017. https://www.ncbi.nlm.nih.gov/pubmed/9815476.

13. Herxheimer, A., and K. J. Petrie. "Melatonin for the Prevention and Treatment of Jet Lag." The Cochrane Database of Systematic Reviews. Accessed June 04, 2017. doi:10.1002/14651858.CD001520.

CHAPTER 9

1. Tiralongo, E., R. A. Lea, S. S. Wee, M. M. Hanna, and L. R. Griffiths. "Randomised, Double Blind, Placebo-Controlled Trial of Echinacea Supplementation in Air Travellers." Evidence-based Complementary and Alternative Medicine : ECAM. December 20, 2012. Accessed June 04, 2017. doi:10.1155/2012/417267.

2. Nordqvist, Christian. "Fish Oils: Health Benefits, Facts, Research." Medical News Today. October 06, 2016. Accessed June 13, 2017. http://www.medicalnewstoday.com/articles/40253.php.

3. Wu, Brian. "Magnesium Glycinate: Uses, Benefits, and Side Effects." Medical News Today. January 22, 2017. Accessed June 13, 2017. http://www.medicalnewstoday.com/articles/315372.php.

4. Aranow, Cynthia. "Vitamin D and the Immune System." Journal of Investigative Medicine : The Official Publication of the American Federation for Clinical Research. August 2011. Accessed June 13, 2017. doi:10.231/JIM.0b013e31821b8755.

5. Greenblatt, James M. "Psychological Consequences of Vitamin D Deficiency." Psychology Today. November 14, 2011. Accessed June 13, 2017. https://www.psychologytoday.com/blog/the-breakthrough-depression-solution/201111/psychological-consequences-vitamin-d-deficiency.

Index

Entries in *italics* denote recipes, in addition to book titles.
Page numbers in *italics* denote illustrations.

A

eggs
    problems with, 71, 85, 90, 202
    as vitamin source, 226, 230
elderberry syrup, 207
electrical nature of bodies, 146-47, 257
electrocardiograms (EKGs), 257
electroencephalogram (EEGs), 257
electromagnetic fields (EMFs), dangers of, 182-83, 191, 271
electronics, problems of, 133, 144, 147, 148, 151, 181, 182-83, 187, 255
elimination (pooping), improvement of, 72, 165-67, 173, 204, 272
elimination diet, 90-97
    acceptable foods for, 71-72, 81, 89, 91, 93-97 (*see also* recipes)
    benefits of, 69, 72-73, 82, 90, 166, 233, 269
    Dr. Alex's Quick Start Guide for, 72, 82, 89, 90-97
    and food sensitivities, 70-71, 90, 92-93, 202, 233
    and leaky gut syndrome, 69, 202
    personal story about, 84-85
    reactionary foods and, 90, 92-93, 202
    resources for, 89
    sample menu plan for, 93-97
emotional freedom technique (EFT) or tapping, 188-89, 191
emotional functioning, 134, 195
emotional stress, 197
    see also stress
emotional toxins
    as cause of chronic stress, 186
    Dr. Alex's best detox tools for, 188-89, 191
    practices for weeding (cleansing), 186-88
    see also stress
endocrine disruptors, 162, 163, 167, 170, 172, 177, 238
energy medicine practices, 257-61
    acupuncture, 245, 259, 263
    being in nature (*see* earthing)
    craniosacral therapy, 260, 263
    definition of, 257
    massage, 149, 156, 185, 245, 260-61
    qigong (tai chi), 258-59
    qoya, 259
    Reiki, 259-60, 263
    yoga, 153, 184, 258, 259
enriching gut health, *see* gut health (step 5)
enteric nervous system, 195
entrees, 76, 116-20
    Buffalo Burger in a Napa Wrap, 94, 119-20
    Grilled Salmon with Pineapple Cilantro Salsa, 95, 118-19
    Ground Beef Picadillo with Lettuce Cups, 97, 116-18
    ideas for, 76, 94-97

H

cleaners, problems with, 178-79, 241
dust, problems with, 181-82
electromagnetic fields, dangers of, 182-83
flame retardants, problems with, 162, 181, 183, 184
in kitchen, 182, 241
and no-shoe policy indoors, 183
and over-sanitizing, 200, 201, 206, 208
see also toxins
"How the Sugar Industry Shifted the Blame to Fat" (O'Conner), 76
hsCRP (lab), 235, 237, 243
hunter-gatherer lifestyle, 66-67, 128
hurried vs. mindful gardener metaphor, 15-19, 24, 262-63, 276
hydrochloric acid (HCL), 203, 220, 222
hydrolyzed grass-fed beef protein powder, 81, 98-104, 122-23, 272
hydrolyzed grass-fed collagen protein powder, 81, 98-104, 122-23, 272
Hyman, Mark, 27-28
hypersensitivity, 68, 242
hypertension, 258
hypnosis, 188
hypothyroidism, 232-33

I

IgE mediated response to food, 68
IgG antibodies, 68, 236, 243
IgG food sensitivity test, 69, 234, 240
immune system
        and alternatives to antibiotics, 206-7, 208
        help for, 69, 81, 109, 201, 206-7, 208, 272
        and inflammation in gut, 68-69, 194-98
        and nutrient interactions, 60
        and stress, 129-30, 196-98
        and vitamin and iron deficiencies, 220, 224-25, 227, 229
        see also autoimmune diseases
inflammation
        as cause of all chronic diseases, 180, 186, 197, 237
        diagnosis, difficulties of, 237
        diagnostic labs for, 237
        and psychobiotics for mental health, pain, 209
        reduction of, 134, 272 (*see also* gut health (step 5))
        stress as cause of, 68-69, 196-98
        toxins as cause of, 180, 186
infrared saunas, 184, 185, 191
Inner Balance (biofeedback tool), 154, 157
insomnia, 93, 128, 146, 148, 229, 237
        see also sleep

K

kale, 107, 115, 121, 168
kefir, 166, 204
kelp, 173
kimchi, 166, 204
kiwi, 168
kombucha, 71-72, 91, 166, 204

L

labs, diagnostic
    advanced, 22, 24, 202, 210, 216-17, 232-41, 242-44
    for autoimmune diseases, 240-41, 242
    for Candida overgrowth, 236-37
    determining need for, 202, 203, 209-10, 214, 216
    for food sensitivities, 69, 234, 240, 243
    for Hashimoto's Disease and thyroid issues, 233, 243-44
    for hormonal imbalances, 238-39
    for inflammation, 237
    for iron deficiency, 221-22, 223
    for leaky gut, 234
    for metabolic disease (blood sugar), 235
    for mycotoxin exposure, 241, 243
    for vitamin B12 deficiency, 225-26, 240, 242
    for vitamin D deficiency, 229, 240
laughter for relaxation, 261
leaky gut syndrome
    chronic inflammation and, 69, 197-201
    diagnosis, difficulties of, 197, 198, 234
    and elimination diet, 69, 202
    explanation of, 68-69
    and food sensitivities, 68-69, 197-98
    help for, 69, 90-97, 109, 197-98
    labs for detecting, 234
    symptoms of, 68-69, 197-200, 218, 234, 235, 236, 237
    see also elimination diet; gut health (step 5)
learning disabilities, 221
leeks, 205
legumes (peanuts), 65, 71, 80, 90, 91, 220
lemon water, 83, 173, 203
leptin, 235
LH (lab), 238
Life in Bloom Facebook group, 55, 73, 88, 89, 277
lifestyles
    of hunter-gatherer, 66-67, 128

causes of, 229, 234-35
diagnostic labs and solutions for, 235
metabolism, 79, 162, 195, 205
methylation, 224-25, 227
methylcobalamin (for vitamin B12), 226
methylmalonic acid test, 225
Mexican cooking methods, 64-65
microbiome, gut, 194-96, 200, 201, 206, 208, 236, 272
micronutrient testing, 241, 243
migraines, 25, 27, 28
"Mindful Gardener" metaphor, 15-19, 24, 262-63, 276
mindfulness
    as counterbalance to stress response, 254-55
    and healthy digestion, 61-62, 188
    principles of practice of, 255-56, 263
    see also meditation
minerals, 60, 65, 98, 172, 203, 204, 218
    see also specific minerals
mistakes, attitude toward, 38, 50
mold, 241-42
Monterey Bay Aquarium's Seafood Watch program, 176
mood, changes in, 22, 72, 92, 198, 199, 209, 241, 260
motivation, see "Why," big
movement
    and benefits of exercise, 184, 185, 235
    vs. exercise, 151, 153
    goals for, 152, 153, 156
    and use of tracking device, 152
MTHFR genetic mutation test, 225, 227, 240
multiple sclerosis, 239
multivitamin, 272
Muscle Activation Technique (MAT™) practitioners, 245
music, use of, 50-51, 133, 141, 142
mycotoxin exposure
    diagnostic testing for, 241, 243
    as underdiagnosed condition, 241-42
myelin sheath, 224

N

National Toxicology Program, 160
natural alternatives to antibiotics, 206-7, 208
nature, being in, 140, 141, 142, 147, 148, 156, 201, 206, 208, 261
naturopaths, 245
nectarines, 167
neurotransmitters, 208, 227

omega-6 fats, 77
Omnivore's Dilemma, The (Pollan), 63
1,4-dioxane, 178
onions, 168, 173, 205
online resources, 39, 58, 89, 157, 190-91, 211, 246, 250, 263, 277
optimism, attitude of, 54, 55, 142
organic acid testing, 243
organic foods, 167-70
Oriental medicine, doctors of, 245
oscillococcinum, 207
osteoporosis, 229
outdoors, being, 140, 141, 142, 147, 148, 156, 201, 206, 208, 261
over-sanitizing, 200, 201, 206, 208

P

pain
    help for, 72, 148, 208-9, 245, 255, 258, 260
    joint, 49, 69, 70, 72, 84, 93, 242
    personal stories about, 49, 84-85
    and psychobiotics, 208-9
    and vitamin D deficiency, 229
palm kernel oil, 78
panic attacks, 25-27, 29, 49, 198
papayas, 168
paranoia, 225
parasympathetic mode, 130, 132, 134, 142, 154
Parkinson's Disease, 162
passionflower tea, 146
patient coordinators, 246-47
Pavlov, Ivan, 61
peaches, 167
peanuts (legumes), 65, 71, 80, 90, 91, 220
pea protein isolate (powder), 80, 81, 98-104, 122-23, 272
pears, 168
peas, sweet (frozen), 168
peppers, 85, 168, 202
perfectionist vs. expansive attitude, 36-38, 39, 54, 56-57, 186-87, 253-54, 268, 277
periods (menstruation), 219, 222
permission slips for healing journey, 36, 39
personal care products and make-up
    non-toxic alternatives for, 177, 191
    as source for toxins, 176, 241
    as water contaminant, 171
personal stories, 24-29, 32-33, 49, 67, 84-85, 136-37, 141, 179, 215-16, 252-53, 265-67
pesticides, 161, 162, 163, 167, 169, 170, 171, 172, 177

purpose of, 131, 156
    steps for creating, 132, 133, 157
sanitizing, excessive, 200, 201, 206, 208
saturated fats, 77, 78
sauerkraut, 166, 204
saunas/steam rooms, 184, 185, 191
scleroderma, 239
seafood, *see* fish and seafood
seaweed, 91, 173
sedentary lifestyle, problems with, 185
"seeds" of desire
    caring for, 53-57
    personal stories about, 49, 265-67
    ritual for sowing, 50-53, 52, 58
    selecting, 20, 42-43, 45-50, 58, 88
    see also intentions
Seed Words, 45-50, 58
self-analysis, *see* "Why," big
self-care
    approaches to, 39, 48, 149, 268
    importance of, 31-34, 198, 206, 210, 274-75
    permission for, 35-36, 57
    see also rooting deeply (step 3)
self-talk, negative, 187
serum ferritin (lab), 221-22
sex drive, 72, 129-30, 232
sex hormone binding globulin (lab), 239
shoes, not for indoors, 183
shortness of breath, 221
showers (hot/cold) for sweating, 184
SIBO (small intestinal bacterial overgrowth), 223, 242, 244
Silent Spring Institute, 178
Sinek, Simon, 58
Sister Alice, 26-27
Sjogren's syndrome, 239
skin
    help for, 72, 81, 83, 102, 170, 172, 184, 185, 191, 272
    irritations of, 93, 197, 199, 232, 237, 241
    and sun exposure, 228, 230, 231, 250
sleep
    amount needed, 144
    and diet, 72, 145
    importance of, 143-44, 156
    improvement of, 72, 134, 144-45, 147, 148, 183, 189, 255
    and insomnia, 93, 128, 146, 148, 229, 237
    natural remedies for, 146, 271, 272
slippery elm bark, 204

swimming, 147, 150, 153
sympathetic autonomic nervous system response, 129
synthetic chemicals, 160-61

T

tampons and pads, 177, 191
tapping or emotional freedom technique (EFT), 188-89, 191
tea, 83, 91, 93-97, 145, 146, 174
Ted Talks, 58
Teflon, dangers of, 182
testosterone (lab), 238
tests, *see* labs, diagnostic
therapeutic touch, 260
therapist, holistic, 245
THINX underwear, 177, 191
thirty-day elimination diet, *see* elimination diet
three-step system for gut health, 202-6
thyroglobulin (TG) antibodies, 233, 244
thyroid function
    causes of problems with, 162, 181, 199, 215-16, 233
    diagnostic tests for, 233, 243-44
    diseases involving, 232-33
    help for, 147, 216
thyroid peroxidase (TPO) antibodies test, 233, 244
tomatoes, 84, 168, 202
tongue, red and swollen, 225
topsoil, depleted, 218
Total Twitch Twitch Training (t3 Approach), 153
toxins
    most common, 163
    types of, 160-63
    see also detoxification (step 4); emotional toxins; household toxins
traditional cooking methods, *see* cooking methods, traditional
transgenerational damage, 65-66, 163
travel challenges, managing, 270-71
trigger foods for gut problems, 70-71, 202-3, 206
TSH, 147, 233, 244
turmeric/curcumin, 207
25-hydroxy vitamin D (25-OH D) test, 229

U

"UCLA Study: Friendships Among Women," 137
ulcerative colitis, 239

Y

yeast infections, overgrowth, 196, 199, 236
yoga, 153, 184, 258, 259
yogurts, 64, 90, 121, 166, 204

Z

zinc, 65, 112, 201, 204, 207
zonulin test, 234, 240, 244

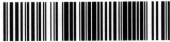

Made in the USA
Columbia, SC
20 October 2018